The Duke Elder Exam of Ophthalmology

A Comprehensive Guide for Success

The Duke Elder Exam of Ophthalmology

A Comprehensive Guide for Success

Edited by

Mostafa Khalil
Junior Doctor, Ninewells Hospital and Medical School
Dundee, Scotland, United Kingdom

Omar Kouli
Medical Student, University of Dundee
Dundee, Scotland, United Kingdom

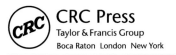

CRC Press
Taylor & Francis Group
Boca Raton London New York

CRC Press is an imprint of the
Taylor & Francis Group, an **informa** business

CRC Press
Taylor & Francis Group
6000 Broken Sound Parkway NW, Suite 300
Boca Raton, FL 33487-2742

© 2020 by Taylor & Francis Group, LLC
CRC Press is an imprint of Taylor & Francis Group, an Informa business

No claim to original U.S. Government works

Printed on acid-free paper

International Standard Book Number-13: 978-0-367-22479-0 (Paperback)

Library of Congress Cataloging-in-Publication Data

Names: Khalil, Mostafa (Of Ninewells Hospital & Medical School), author, editor. | Kouli, Omar, author, editor.
Title: The Duke Elder Exam of ophthalmology : a comprehensive guide for success / authors, Mostafa Khalil, Omar Kouli.
Description: Boca Raton : Taylor & Francis, 2020. | Includes bibliographical references and index.
Identifiers: LCCN 2019008177| ISBN 9780367224790 (pbk. : alk. paper) | ISBN 9780429275081 (ebook)
Subjects: | MESH: Eye Diseases | Ocular Physiological Phenomena | Examination Question | Study Guide
Classification: LCC RE49 | NLM WW 18.2 | DDC 617.70076--dc23
LC record available at https://lccn.loc.gov/2019008177

Visit the Taylor & Francis Web site at
http://www.taylorandfrancis.com

and the CRC Press Web site at
http://www.crcpress.com

Dedication

We dedicate this book to our parents, who have been very supportive and have encouraged and inspired us throughout the entire process. Thank you, Dr Mohamed Khalil and Dr Sahar Hussein. Thank you, Dr Oussama Kouli and Mrs Kinana Hammour.

Contents

Preface

Sir William Stewart Duke-Elder (22 April 1898–27 March 1978) was a Scottish ophthalmologist widely referred to as the "Father of Ophthalmology" for his significant impact on the field during his era. He was born and raised in the city of Dundee, completed his education at the University of St Andrews and went on to produce seven volumes of the *Textbook of Ophthalmology* and fifteen volumes of the *System of Ophthalmology*, as well as many others.

The Duke Elder Exam, named for Sir William Stewart Duke-Elder, is a competitive national undergraduate prize examination, which is challenging and demanding. Nonetheless, the exam is rewarding as it is filled with incentives in the form of three awards: (1) top 10%, (2) top 20 performing candidates, and finally, (3) top performing candidate. Each of these awards gives the successful candidate two valuable points towards their specialty application.

The format of the exam is 90 multiple choice questions (MCQs) covering clinical ophthalmology, basic sciences, anatomy and optics.

There is currently no comprehensive textbook that covers the Duke Elder curriculum in its entirety. This volume fills this gap and is the first that provides an in-depth educational resource. It includes a basic sciences chapter, subspecialty clinical chapters that begin with anatomy, and ends with two 90 MCQ question banks to test the student's knowledge.

Authored by two previous successful candidates from the University of Dundee, edited by a specialist ophthalmic trainee who was also previously a successful candidate (third in the UK) and two consultant ophthalmologists, this book will assist the candidate in maximizing their performance and achieving their desired goals.

Mostafa Khalil
Omar Kouli

Acknowledgements

We thank the publishers Taylor & Francis/CRC Press, and in particular Shivangi Pramanik, commissioning editor, and Himani Dwivedi, editorial assistant, for their help and support throughout this project. We are grateful to the ophthalmic imaging team at Ninewells Hospital, and in particular Mr James Talbot, ophthalmic photographer, for providing us with photographs of ocular conditions to aid visual understanding of conditions. We thank Dr Yeeling Wong for her design of the front cover of the book. We also thank Ms Tasnim Kouli for her artistic drawings and diagrams throughout the book. Finally, we thank Mr Ahmed Khogali for his efforts in reviewing the grammar of the book.

Editors

Mostafa Khalil is a Foundation Doctor at Ninewells Hospital and Medical School in the United Kingdom. He graduated from the University of Dundee in Scotland with the following awards: MBChB, George Ranken Tudhope Prize: Preparation in Practice, Doctor as a Scholar and Scientist for Highest Grade in Medical School Finals Exam 2017, Dr AR Moodie Prize in Ophthalmology for being the highest-performing candidate in ophthalmology during medical school, and a special commendation from the president of the Royal College of Ophthalmologists for placing fifth in the UK (out of 370 candidates) on the Duke Elder Exam 2018.

Omar Kouli is a fourth-year medical student at the University of Dundee, Scotland at the time of this writing. During his university career he has thus far been awarded with the following prizes: winner of the National Undergraduate Neuroanatomy Competition 2018, and a special commendation from the president of the Royal College of Ophthalmologists for placing fourth in the UK (out of 370 candidates) on the Duke Elder Exam 2018.

Contributors

Nemat Ahmed
Medical Student
University of Dundee
Dundee, Scotland, United Kingdom

Stewart Gillan
Consultant Ophthalmologist
Ninewells Hospital
Dundee, Scotland, United Kingdom

Ahmed Hassane
Medical Student
University of Dundee
Dundee, Scotland, United Kingdom

Bilal Ibrahim
Foundation Doctor
Ninewells Hospital
Dundee, Scotland, United Kingdom

Mostafa Khalil
Junior Doctor
Ninewells Hospital and Medical School
Dundee, Scotland, United Kingdom

Tarek Khalil
Foundation Doctor
Ninewells Hospital
Dundee, Scotland, United Kingdom

Omar Kouli
Medical Student
University of Dundee
Dundee, Scotland, United Kingdom

Obaid Kousha
Specialty Registrar
Ninewells Hospital
Dundee, Scotland, United Kingdom

Rizwan Malik
Consultant Ophthalmologist
King Khaled Eye Specialist Hospital
Riyadh, Saudi Arabia

Exam format

The Duke Elder Prize Examination is a national ophthalmology exam in the UK hosted annually by the Royal College of Ophthalmologists. All current UK medical students are eligible to sit the exam.

It is a 2-hour written exam, with 90 MCQs. Most of the questions are clinically based; however, a significant portion comes from basic science and socioeconomic and miscellaneous topics relevant to ophthalmology.

The clinical topics broken down by the Royal College are from the following subspecialties:

- Cornea and external eye disease
- Cataracts
- Glaucoma
- Medical retina and vitreoretinal surgery
- Strabismus and paediatric ophthalmology
- Neuro-ophthalmology
- Ocular adnexal and orbital disease
- Refractive errors and optics

The deadline to register for the exam is usually in December each year and the exam takes place in early March. Please refer to the Royal College of Ophthalmologists website for more information, as it may change from year to year.

Author tips

The Duke Elder Exam is a national undergraduate exam. It is notoriously difficult in comparison to medical school level ophthalmology exams. It can best be described as a bridge between postgraduate and undergraduate examinations, meant to filter out those dedicated to the specialty.

Preparation can be daunting, and so students should plan to give themselves approximately 3 months to maximize their efforts, especially while balancing other university commitments. Our key advice is to not be discouraged if you forget a topic you previously learned. Think back to starting medical school, and how overwhelming it may have seemed with all the new terms you had to adjust to, yet you were still able to overcome such obstacles; the Duke Elder Exam is no different.

As stated by the Royal College of Ophthalmologists, the exam is intended for medical students who have completed their ophthalmology blocks in their undergraduate curriculum. We have followed that advice and so this book will assume a basic level of understanding of the eye. It may be worthwhile to watch some videos of the basic anatomy of the eye before starting this book, especially if you have not covered ophthalmology in your university yet.

Our tips on how to effectively use this book are as follows:

1. Start with the first chapter, 'Basic Science, Investigations and Lasers'. Following this, it will be useful to refer back to the relevant sections of this chapter as you approach the clinical chapters. For example, in Chapter 12 on glaucoma, it will be useful to look back to the basic science chapter and review the mechanisms of the drugs used to treat glaucoma.
2. Each clinical chapter starts with anatomy. Again, it will be useful to refer back to the relevant anatomy when studying certain eye conditions that require anatomical knowledge.
3. Each section in this book is relevant to the Duke Elder Exam – do not skip over topics! The Duke Elder Exam requires a wide base of knowledge, which includes topics that may not seem particularly relevant to you as a medical student. For example, laser safety, different sutures or socioeconomic topics such as Vision 2020 may not be taught as part of your undergraduate syllabus, but the Duke Elder Exam is designed to test your understanding beyond the standards of medical school.

4. Use the questions at the end to test your knowledge. These questions have been developed at the level appropriate for the Duke Elder Exam.
5. Read the book more than once. The information will become easier to grasp and you will gain an even deeper understanding of what is being discussed.

The bottom line is, work hard, do not take shortcuts, do not give up, and ignore any doubts you may have or that have been expressed by others. If you stay dedicated, you will be successful.

1

Basic science, investigations and lasers

TAREK KHALIL, BILAL IBRAHIM, STEWART GILLAN
AND OBAID KOUSHA

1.1 EMBRYOLOGIC ORIGINS OF EYE STRUCTURES

Ocular structures are derived from the germ layers described in Table 1.1.

1.2 GENETICS

In this section, basic knowledge of chromosomes and types of inheritance are covered, along with examples of conditions and their associated inheritance (Table 1.2).

1.2.1 Chromosomes

Eukaryotic cells differ from primitive cells with the presence of the nucleus. Deoxyribonucleic acid (DNA) is present in the nucleus and carries genetic information needed for cell production. The DNA molecules are packaged into structures called chromosomes.

Table 1.1 Summary of ocular structures' embryologic origins

Germ layer	Ocular structures
Surface ectoderm	Conjunctival and corneal epithelium
	Nasolacrimal duct
	Lens
	Lacrimal gland
	Eyelids
Neuroectoderm	Neurosensory retina
	Pigment epithelium of the retina, iris and ciliary body
	Pupillary sphincter and dilator muscles
	Optic nerve
Neural crest	Corneal endothelium
	Trabecular meshwork
	Stroma of cornea, iris and ciliary body
	Ciliary muscle
	Choroid
	Sclera
	Orbital cartilage and bone
Mesoderm	Extraocular muscles
	Blood vessels
	Schlemm's canal endothelium
	Sclera (temporal portion)

Chromosomes have a short arm, denoted as 'p', and a long arm, denoted as 'q'. Human cells contain 46 chromosomes: 22 identical pairs and a pair of sex chromosomes. Genetic information can be carried on any of these chromosomes, and hence inheritance can be autosomal or sex-linked (X-linked). Other forms of inheritance that are covered here include mitochondrial inheritance, which is passed only by the mother.

1.2.2 Inheritance

In autosomal recessive (AR) conditions, an offspring needs to inherit both alleles of a faulty gene to express the condition, otherwise, they are phenotypically normal and called carriers of the gene. The opposite is true of autosomal dominant (AD) conditions, where an offspring needs only one faulty allele to express the condition.

X-linked inheritance is slightly different. Genes are passed from the sex chromosomes. Females have two X chromosomes while males have an X and Y chromosome. This means that a mother will always pass on an X chromosome while a father will either pass a Y chromosome (to a son) or an X chromosome (to a daughter) to their offspring. Faulty genes are usually expressed on the X chromosome.

Table 1.2 Inheritance of ocular and systemic pathologies

Inheritance	Conditions
AD	Congenital cataracts
	Best disease
	Fuchs' corneal dystrophy (also sporadic)
	Granular and lattice corneal dystrophies
	Marfan syndrome
	Neurofibromatosis
	Retinitis pigmentosa (also AR or XLR)
	Retinoblastoma (most commonly sporadic)
	Stickler syndrome
	Tuberous sclerosis
	Von Hippel-Lindau (VHL)
AR	Congenital glaucoma (most commonly sporadic)
	Oculocutaneous albinism
	Stargardt disease
	Retinitis pigmentosa-like conditions
XLR	Fabry disease
	Lowe syndrome
	Ocular albinism
	Retinoschisis
XLD	Alport syndrome (also AR)
Mitochondrial	Kearns-Sayre syndrome
	Leber hereditary optic neuropathy

In X-linked recessive (XLR) conditions, a male offspring will only be affected if his mother is affected. A female is affected if both parents are affected but is a carrier if only one of the parents is affected. In X-linked dominant (XLD) conditions, the same concepts apply for the male child; that is, males can only inherit the condition from their mother. However, a female can express the condition from her father alone even if her mother is unaffected.

1.3 MICROBIOLOGY

In this section, microorganisms and the function of antibiotics/antifungals are discussed. It is best to refer back to this section when coming across an organism causing a specific ocular disease to appreciate it better.

1.3.1 Bacteria

Bacteria are unicellular prokaryotic organisms that contain DNA and ribonucleic acid (RNA) freely in the cytoplasm. Reproduction is via a process called

Table 1.3 Classification of bacteria

		Gram positive	Gram negative
Cocci	Aerobic	Clusters: *Staphylococcus aureus* (coagulase +ve) and *S. epidermidis* (coagulase −ve)	*Neisseria gonorrhoeae* and *meningitides* (diplococci)
	Anaerobic	Chains: *Streptococcus* spp. (facultative)	N/A
Bacilli	Aerobic	Spore forming: *Bacillus cereus*	*Haemophilus influenzae* and *Pseudomonas aeruginosa*
	Anaerobic	Spore forming: *Clostridium* sp. Non-spore forming: *Propionibacterium acne* Filamentous: *Actinomyces israelii*	*Campylobacter* sp.

binary fission. Bacteria can be classified according to their morphology and gram staining (Table 1.3). Bacteria have various characteristics:

1. Cell wall: Gram-positive bacterial cell walls are predominantly made of peptidoglycan (stains purple), while Gram-negative bacteria is predominantly made of an outer plasma membrane (stains pink).
2. Cell membrane.
3. Plasmids (fragments of DNA): Thought to be the reason behind antibiotic resistance.
4. Flagella: Helps with motility.
5. Pili: Transfers DNA between bacteria.
6. Exotoxins and endotoxin: In Gram-positive and Gram-negative bacteria, respectively.

OTHER BACTERIA

1. Mycobacteria: Acid-fast bacilli that are aerobic and non-spore forming. They contain a cell wall that does not allow Gram staining; Ziehl-Neelson stain is used.
2. Chlamydia: Obligate intracellular bacterium. They can exist in the form of either elementary bodies (infectious) or reticular bodies (found in host cells only) during their life cycle.

1.3.2 Fungus

Fungi are eukaryotic organisms that reproduce sexually. They can be classified into three broad groups, as follows.

YEASTS

Yeasts are unicellular microorganisms. A good example is *Candida albicans*. Candida is a commensal that reproduces by budding. It causes infection in immunocompromised patients and is the most common cause of endogenous endophthalmitis presenting with white fluffy retinal lesions.

FILAMENTOUS

Their cells grow in a branching-like pattern. *Aspergillus* spp. and *Fusarium* spp. are types of filamentous fungi. They are common in warm climates and can cause fungal keratitis, usually following ocular trauma.

DIMORPHIC

These fungi have properties of both yeasts and filamentous fungi. *Histoplasma capsulatum* is a soil fungus, endemic in Mississippi and Ohio River Valleys. Transmission is via inhalation. It can cause presumed ocular histoplasmosis syndrome (POHS).

1.3.3 Protozoa and helminth

Protozoa are single-celled eukaryotic parasites. Helminth are parasitic worms that can cause infection.

EXAMPLES OF OCULAR-RELATED INFECTIONS

1. *Toxoplasma gondii*: Obligate intracellular parasite (protozoa). Cats are the definitive host. Transmission to humans is via fecal-oral spread, inhalation or undercooked meats. It can also be transmitted in pregnancy via vertical transmission. *T. gondii* can cause congenital or adult toxoplasmosis.
2. *Acanthamoeba*: Protozoa that can be found in soil, water or swimming pools. It can cause severe keratitis.
3. *Toxocara*: A helminth nematode (roundworm). Their hosts are cats and dogs. It can be transmitted to humans through fecal-contaminated material. It causes toxocariasis which presents with endophthalmitis in children.
4. *Onchocerca volvulus*: The most common helminth-related ocular infection. The vectors are Simulium blackflies. It causes onchocerciasis ('river blindness') and is endemic in Africa.

1.3.4 Viruses

Viruses are acellular parasites that require cellular material from other organisms to replicate. A virus consists of DNA or RNA enclosed in a protein known as a capsid. DNA viruses produce intranuclear inclusions, while RNA viruses produce intracytoplasmic inclusions.

DNA VIRUSES

- Herpes simplex virus (HSV)
- Varicella zoster virus (VZV)

- Cytomegalovirus (CMV): A very weak virus and only infects immunocompromised patients with a CD4$^+$ count $<$50
- Epstein-Barr virus (EBV)
- Adenovirus
- *Molluscum contagiosum*

RNA VIRUSES

- Measles, mumps and rubella
- HIV

1.3.5 Antibiotics/antifungals

Antibiotics or antifungals work by affecting the cell wall, cell membrane, protein or nucleic acid synthesis (Table 1.4).

Table 1.4 Antibiotics/antifungals mechanism of action

Mechanism of action	Examples
Inhibits cell wall synthesis	Penicillin
	Cephalosporin
	Vancomycin
Inhibits cell membrane function	Antifungals: Imidazoles, amphotericin and nystatin
Inhibits protein synthesis	Aminoglycosides
	Tetracyclines
	Erythromycin
	Chloramphenicol
Inhibits nucleic acid synthesis	Fluoroquinolones (DNA gyrase)
	Metronidazole

1.4 IMMUNOLOGY

1.4.1 Innate versus adaptive immunity

The innate immune system refers to a rapid nonspecific response of the immune system towards a foreign antigen. Neutrophils, macrophages, dendritic cells and the complement system are part of the innate system.

The adaptive immune system refers to an immune response towards a specific antigen, mediated by lymphocytes (T and B cells).

1.4.2 Major histocompatibility complex

Major histocompatibility complex (MHC), also called human leucocyte antigen (HLA) in humans (Table 1.5), are found on the short arm of chromosome 6. They have an important function in antigen recognition by presenting self and pathogenic peptide fragments for identification by T cells.

Table 1.5 Ocular and systemic associations with HLA subtypes

HLA subtypes	Conditions
HLA-A29	Birdshot choroidopathy
HLA-A11	Sympathetic ophthalmia
HLA-B7	Presumed ocular histoplasmosis syndrome (POHS)
HLA-B22	Vogt-Koyanagi-Harada syndrome (VKH)
HLA-B27	Psoriatic arthritis
	Ankylosing spondylitis
	Reactive arthritis
	Enteropathic arthritis
HLA-B51	Behçet disease
HLA-BW5	Posner-Schlossman syndrome
HLA-DR2	Pars planitis
	POHS
	Multiple sclerosis
HLA-DR4	Sympathetic ophthalmia
	Rheumatoid arthritis
	VKH
HLA-DR5	Juvenile idiopathic arthritis
HLA-DR15	Multiple sclerosis (MS)

MHC-1 (HLA-A, HLA-B, HLA-C) are expressed on all cells and stimulate CD8+ cytotoxic T cells. MHC-2 (HLA-DR, HLA-DP, HLA-DQ) stimulate CD4+ T-helper cells and are expressed on specialized antigen-presenting cells such as macrophages.

1.4.3 Cytokines

Cytokines are molecules responsible for recruitment and proliferation of the innate and adaptive immune systems. They include the following.

TUMOUR NECROSIS FACTOR

Tumour necrosis factor (TNF)-alpha are proinflammatory cells produced by macrophages. They help in the activation and differentiation of immune cells and increase vascular permeability. They are therefore mediators of inflammation and septic shock.

INTERLEUKINS

Interleukins (ILs) mediate communication between different cells and are important in regulating immune responses. There are various types of IL; key examples are:

- IL-1: Induces immune responses and causes fever
- IL-2: Proliferation of T and B cells
- IL-5: Regulates growth and activation of eosinophils

- IL-6: Involved in differentiation of B cells and production of c-reactive protein (CRP); causes fever
- IL-8: Attracts neutrophils, T cells, basophils and eosinophils
- IL-10: Suppresses immune cells
- IL-12: Differentiates T cells into TH1 and enhances cytotoxicity

CHEMOKINES

Involved in chemotaxis.

INTERFERONS

Interferons act as proinflammatory or immunomodulatory cells. They can be also thought of as antiviral agents. Interferon beta can be used in managing multiple sclerosis (MS).

1.5 DRUG MECHANISMS AND SIDE EFFECTS

1.5.1 Glaucoma and intraocular pressure

Normal intraocular pressure (IOP) within a population is considered to be within ± 2 standard deviations of the mean IOP, which ranges between 10 and 21 mmHg. IOP increases with age and follows a circadian rhythm, with the highest IOP recorded in the morning. IOP in normal individuals has an average diurnal fluctuation ranging between 2 and 6 mmHg, while glaucoma patients have a higher diurnal fluctuation (>10 mmHg). Elevated IOP can cause glaucoma if left untreated.

IOP-RAISING AGENTS

- Steroids
- Tropicamide (close-angle glaucoma)
- Ketamine

IOP-LOWERING AGENTS

These are primarily used in managing glaucoma (Table 1.6). Uncommon drugs that can lower IOP include:

- Cannabinoids: Short-lasting effect and tachyphylaxis (reduced response to the drug over time)
- Alcohol: Transient effect on IOP

1.5.2 Cataracts

Drugs causing lens opacification and cataracts include:

- Steroids
- Amiodarone
- Allopurinol
- Chlorpromazine
- Tobacco smoke

Table 1.6 IOP-lowering medications

Drug	Mechanism	Side effects
Beta-blockers (e.g. timolol)	Decrease aqueous production	Decreased corneal sensation, dry eye, tachyphylaxis, bradycardia, bronchospasm and nocturnal hypotension
Prostaglandin analogue (e.g. latanoprost)	Increase aqueous drainage via the uveoscleral outflow	Conjunctival hyperaemia, iris hyperpigmentation, increased eyelash length and cystoid macular oedema (CMO)
Alpha-2 agonists (e.g. apraclonidine)	Decrease aqueous production and increase uveoscleral outflow	Follicular conjunctivitis, contact dermatitis, tachyphylaxis, dry mouth and sedation. Used with caution in infants as they can cross the blood-brain barrier
Topical carbonic anhydrase inhibitors (CAI) (e.g. dorzolamide)	Decrease aqueous production	Ocular stinging, bitter taste and punctate keratitis. Contraindicated in patients with sulphonamide allergies
Systemic CAI (e.g. acetazolamide)	Similar to topical CAI	Paraesthesia, urine frequency (diuretic effect), hypokalaemia, Steven-Johnson syndrome and metabolic acidosis
Miotics (e.g. pilocarpine)	Parasympathomimetics that increase aqueous drainage via trabecular meshwork by causing contraction of ciliary muscles	Myopia, brow ache, miosis and retinal detachment
Osmotic agents (e.g. mannitol)	Lowers IOP by decreasing vitreous volume	Cardiovascular overload

1.5.3 Retina

There are a number of drugs that can have adverse effects on the retina, each presenting with different retinal lesions:

- Cystoid macular oedema: Latanoprost, epinephrine, rosiglitazone and nicotinic acid
- Bull's-eye maculopathy (Figure 1.1): Hydroxychloroquine and chloroquine
- Crystalline maculopathy: Tamoxifen

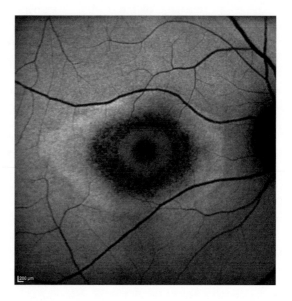

Figure 1.1 Illustration of bull's-eye maculopathy on fundus autofluorescence.

1.5.4 Optic neuropathy

The following drugs have the potential to cause optic nerve damage:

- Ethambutol
- Chloramphenicol
- Amiodarone
- Vigabatrin: Causes binasal visual field defects
- Isoniazid

1.5.5 Vortex keratopathy (corneal verticillata)

This refers to the deposition of asymptomatic grey opacities in a vortex pattern on the corneal epithelium. Causes include:

- Drugs: Amiodarone, chloroquines, indomethacin and phenothiazines.
- Fabry disease: An XLR condition characterised by a deficiency of alpha-galactosidase A. Other features of the disease include burning pain in the extremities, angiokeratomas, renal failure and posterior subcapsular cataracts.

1.6 INVESTIGATIONS

1.6.1 Cornea

KERATOMETRY

Measures the anterior corneal surface curvature.

CORNEAL TOPOGRAPHY

Measures and quantifies the curvature of the whole cornea and provides information on its shape. It uses placido-disc systems which project concentric rings of light on the anterior corneal surface. Indications include keratoconus, astigmatism, laser eye surgery and contact lens fitting.

ULTRASONIC PACHYMETRY

Can be used to measure the central corneal thickness (CCT) using an ultrasonic probe. Normal CCT is between 530 and 545 μm.

1.6.2 Retina

OCULAR COHERENCE TOMOGRAPHY

The ocular coherence tomography (OCT) imaging method uses near-infrared waves through the pupil to the retina to produce a cross-sectional and three-dimensional image of the retina (Figure 1.2). Its main indication is to diagnose and monitor the progression of macular and optic diseases.

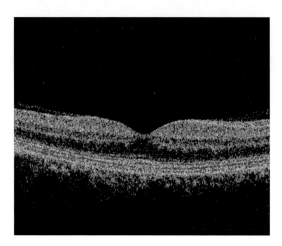

Figure 1.2 Normal OCT image.

FLUORESCENCE ANGIOGRAPHY

In fluorescence angiography (FA), sodium fluorescence, a dye, absorbs blue light (wavelength 465–490 nm) and emits a yellow-green light (530 nm). It is injected into a peripheral vein to circulate to the eye. It passes through the short posterior ciliary artery into the choriocapillaris about 8–12 seconds post-injection and then enters the retinal circulation a second later. Side effects include urine discolouration, nausea, vasovagal syncope, anaphylaxis (rare) and it is contraindicated in shellfish allergy.

In FA, a fundus camera with cobalt blue excitation and yellow-green barrier filters is used to capture several images of the retina during the passage of the dye in the posterior segment of the eye (Figure 1.3) to help detect any vascular abnormalities.

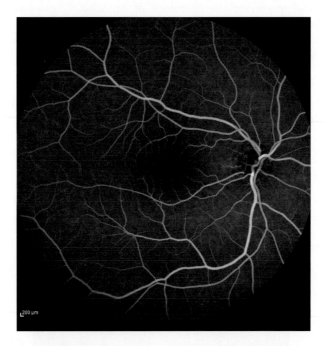

Figure 1.3 Normal FA image.

INDOCYANINE GREEN ANGIOGRAPHY

Indocyanine green (ICG) is 98% bound to albumin in the plasma and has little leakage (low permeability) while passing through the choroid. ICG angiography, unlike FFA, uses near-infrared light. Those factors allow it to visualize the choroid vasculature better (Figure 1.4). Contraindicated in pregnancy and with seafood and iodine allergies.

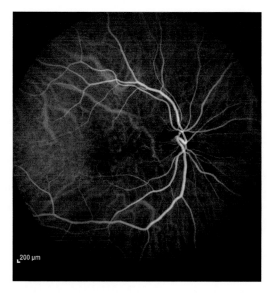

Figure 1.4 Normal ICG angiography image.

FUNDUS AUTOFLUORESCENCE

This technique does not use a dye; however, it detects lipofuscin already present within the retinal pigmented epithelium (RPE) (Figure 1.5). It can be used in Best disease and for monitoring geographic atrophy.

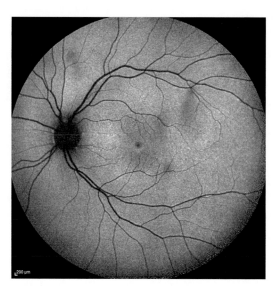

Figure 1.5 Normal fundus autofluorescence image.

ELECTRODIAGNOSTIC TESTS

Electroretinogram (ERG) tests the electrical activity of the retina in response to a light stimulus. Electro-oculogram (EOG) reflects the activity of photoreceptors and RPE; thus retinal diseases proximal to the photoreceptors give normal EOG readings. ERG and EOG may be useful in aiding diagnosis in conditions such as Best disease and retinitis pigmentosa.

1.6.3 Glaucoma

Patients with suspected glaucoma should be examined and investigated to detect and differentiate between different types of glaucoma. This involves measuring the IOP, assessing the iridocorneal angle, measuring the CCT and evaluating the optic nerve head and visual fields.

TONOMETRY

Tonometry is a procedure used to measure IOP. Goldmann applanation tonometry is the most widely used. It follows the Imbert-Fick law to establish the amount of force required to flatten a corneal area of 3.06 mm in diameter assuming a CCT of 520 μm. Factors leading to incorrect measurements include:

- Excessive fluorescein: Overestimates IOP
- Low or high CCT: Underestimates or overestimates IOP, respectively
- Astigmatism
- Calibration errors

GONIOSCOPY

Gonioscopy is used to determine whether the iridocorneal angle is open or closed. Several angle structures exist, and visualization of all structures indicates a wide-open angle, whereas the inability to visualize any structures indicates a closed angle. Those structures, anteriorly to posteriorly, are:

- Schwalbe line
- Nonpigmented trabecular meshwork
- Pigmented trabecular meshwork: Pigmentation is not present at birth and increases with age, mainly following puberty
- Scleral spur: An anterior protrusion of the sclera that marks the attachments of the ciliary body's longitudinal fibres
- Ciliary body

PERIMETRY

Perimetry is used to detect visual field defects and is commonly used in glaucoma and neuro-ophthalmic conditions. Examples of perimetry include Humphrey visual field analysis or Goldmann visual field testing.

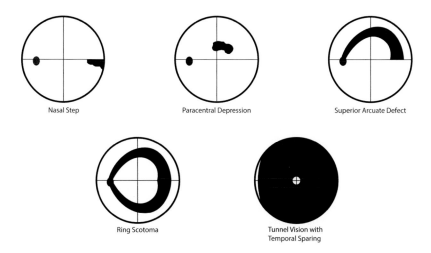

Figure 1.6 Glaucomatous field defects.

Glaucomatous field defects (Figure 1.6) include:

- Nasal step
- Paracentral depressions: Most commonly superonasally
- Arcuate defects: Combination of paracentral depressions
- Ring scotoma: Superior + inferior arcuate defects
- Tunnel vision with a temporal sparing of visual field

1.6.4 Neuro-ophthalmology and orbit

MAGNETIC RESONANCE IMAGING

Magnetic resonance imaging (MRI) scans are produced by the alignment of the hydrogen atoms to the magnetic field around the patient. MRI is useful to aid in the diagnosis of intracranial lesions affecting the visual pathway.

COMPUTED TOMOGRAPHY

Computed tomography (CT) scans utilise a series of x-ray beams to form a detailed image of the body with the aid of a computer. They produce images much faster than an MRI and thus are valuable in acute settings. Common indications include orbital fractures, orbital cellulitis, thyroid eye disease and cerebral haemorrhages. CT angiography is also important to investigate for subarachnoid haemorrhage and intracranial aneurysms, for example, in cases of third nerve palsy.

1.7 LASERS

Light beams emitted by different types of lasers have three fundamental properties: coherency (all emitted photons are in the same phase), monochromaticity (single wavelength) and collimation (narrow with minimal divergence).

Lasers are constructed using three principal parts:

- A source of energy: Light or electrical.
- A medium: Containing atoms or molecules that undergo stimulated emission and is the major determinant of the wavelength. They can be in the form of:
  - Gas (e.g. argon, krypton, carbon dioxide)
  - Liquid (e.g. dyes)
  - Solid (e.g. neodymium-doped yttrium aluminium garnet [Nd:YAG] crystals)
- An optical resonator that uses mirrors to amplify light.

1.7.1 Laser safety

Lasers damage various ocular structures, depending on the wavelength used. For example, ultraviolet light can cause photochemical injuries to the lens and cornea, infrared can cause thermal burns to the lens and cornea, near-infrared can cause thermal burns to the lens and retina and visible light has the potential to cause retinal burns (1).

Lasers are classified into four main groups by the International Electro-technical Commission 60825-1 (2), according to their hazardous effects on the human body. Class 1 is harmless to the eye, while class 4 causes the most harm. Most devices and therapeutic lasers used in ophthalmology fall into classes 3B and 4. Safety measures should be employed to protect the eyes when working with such lasers.

1.7.2 Laser effects and clinical application

Different structures or molecules within the body will react differently to lasers depending on the wavelength of the laser emission. For example:

- Melanin: Found mainly in the RPE and choroid. It absorbs most of the visible spectrum and infrared wavelengths.
- Xanthophyll: Present at the macula. Absorbs blue light (450–495 nm).
- Haemoglobin: Absorbs blue, green (495–570 nm) and yellow light (570–590 nm).

Laser-tissue interaction occurs mainly in the following three ways.

PHOTOTHERMAL

Photovaporization: Vaporization of water from tissues occurs in types of lasers such as carbon dioxide lasers, as they raise the temperature beyond 100°C.
Photocoagulation: Absorption of laser emissions by tissues causes a rise in temperature, leading to protein denaturation. Panretinal photocoagulation (PRP) used in diabetic retinopathy is a good example. Types of photocoagulative lasers include:

- Argon blue-green: Absorbed by melanin, haemoglobin and xanthophyll. Thus it is not used on the macula.

- Krypton red (647 nm): Absorbed by melanin.
- Frequency-doubled Nd:YAG (532 nm): Absorbed by haemoglobin and melanin in the RPE and trabecular meshwork.
- Diode (810 nm): Emits near-infrared radiation and is absorbed by melanin.

PHOTOCHEMICAL

These work by breaking chemical bonds that hold tissue together using ultraviolet light, in a process called photoablation. An excimer laser is a laser that causes photoablation and has important uses in refractive surgery:

- Photorefractive keratectomy (PRK): Corneal epithelium is first removed, then laser ablation is used to reshape the cornea.
- Laser-assisted in situ keratomileusis (LASIK): A corneal flap is created; the stroma is then ablated (to reshape the cornea) and the flap is replaced.
- Laser epithelial keratomileusis (LASEK): The corneal epithelium is peeled using 20% ethanol, laser ablation is performed and the epithelium is replaced.

PHOTO-IONIZING

This type of laser causes destruction of tissues by altering the stable state between photons and electrons. An important example of photo-ionizing lasers includes Nd:YAG (1064 nm), which is used in posterior capsulotomy for treating posterior capsular opacification (PCO) and in peripheral iridotomy used in managing angle-closure glaucoma.

1.8 MISCELLANEOUS

1.8.1 Visual impairment registration

Patients with visual impairment can be registered as either severely sight impaired (blind) or sight impaired (partial visual impairment) according to the criteria set by the Department of Health UK (3):

SEVERELY SIGHT IMPAIRED
- Visual acuity (VA) <3/60 Snellen.
- VA 3/60–6/60 with reduction in visual field (VF).
- VA >6/60 with significantly reduced VF (e.g. inferior altitudinal defects or bitemporal hemianopia).

SIGHT IMPAIRED
- VA 3/60–6/60, with full VF.
- VA 6/60–6/24 with moderate reduction of VF.
- VA ≥6/18 with significant reduction of VF (e.g. homonymous hemianopia).

1.8.2 Driver & Vehicle Licensing Agency (DVLA) driving regulations

THE DVLA CRITERIA FOR CAR AND MOTORCYCLE DRIVERS (4):

1. Ability to read a car registration plate (post-September 2001) at a distance of 20 metres, using corrective glasses or contact lenses if needed.
2. VA $\geq$ 6/12 with both eyes open, or one eye if monocular.
3. VF of at least 120° on the horizontal with extension of at least 50° to the right and left. No significant defect encroaching 20° of fixation above or below the horizontal meridian should be present.

SPECIFIC CASES THAT MUST BE NOTIFIED TO THE DVLA (4):

- Diplopia: Patients may resume driving after confirmation that diplopia is controlled.
- VF defects: Such as retinitis pigmentosa, bilateral glaucoma or bi-temporal hemianopia.
- Nyctalopia.
- Blepharospasm: Even if treated, patients with severe blepharospasm are usually not licenced to drive. Mild cases may be licenced.

1.8.3 Sutures

Choosing a suture material for different ocular structures (Table 1.7) relies on the suture's properties. For example, polyglactin 910 (VICRYL®) and polyglycolic acid (DEXON®) are types of absorbable suture, whereas silk, nylon and polypropylene (PROLENE®) are nonabsorbable.

Table 1.7 Sutures used for ocular structures

Suture	Ocular structure
Silk	Eyelids and sclera
Polyglactin 910	Conjunctiva, muscles and cornea
Nylon	Cornea, sclera and limbus
Polypropylene	Iris
Polyglycolic acid	Limbus

1.8.4 Vision 2020

Vision 2020 was established by the International Agency of the Prevention of Blindness (5) and supported by the World Health Organization (WHO) (6) to eliminate preventable causes of blindness by the year 2020. The following conditions are in their current objectives:

- Cataract: The most common cause of blindness in the world.
- Trachoma: The most common cause of infectious blindness.

- Onchocerciasis: The second most common cause of infectious blindness.
- Refractive errors: The most common cause of visual impairment.
- Childhood blindness: Vitamin A deficiency (the most common cause of nutritional blindness in Africa), measles, retinopathy of prematurity (ROP) and cataract.

REFERENCES

1. Sliney DH, Mellerio J. Effects of optical radiation on the eye. In: Wolbarsht M (editor). *Safety with Lasers and Other Optical Sources: A Comprehensive Handbook.* 1st ed. US: Springer; 1980: 101–59.
2. International Electrotechnical Commission. *60825-1: Safety of Laser Products – Part 1: Equipment Classification and Requirements.* 3rd ed. 2014. https://webstore.iec.ch/publication/3587
3. Department of Health UK. Certificate of Vision Impairment: Explanatory Notes for Consultant Ophthalmologists and Hospital Eye Clinic Staff in England. August 2017. https://assets.publishing.service.gov.uk/government/uploads/system/uploads/attachment_data/file/637590/CVI_guidance.pdf
4. Driving and Vehicle Licensing Agency. Assessing fitness to drive: A guide for medical professionals. August 2018. https://www.gov.uk
5. The International Agency for the Prevention of Blindness. Vision 2020: The Right to Sight. https://www.iapb.org/vision-2020/
6. World Health Organization. Blindness: Vision 2020 – Control of major blinding diseases and disorders. https://www.who.int/mediacentre/factsheets/fs214/en/

2

Optics and refractive errors

NEMAT AHMED, OMAR KOULI, MOSTAFA KHALIL
AND OBAID KOUSHA

2.1 HOW DO WE SEE?

The first step to sight is focusing light onto the fovea of the eye. This process depends on three main things:

1. A clear view to the retina.
2. The length of the eye.
3. The power, measured in diopters (D), of the refractive components of the eye, mainly the cornea (40D) and lens (20D).

2.1.1 Length of the eye

- Axial length of the eyeball is measured from the corneal surface to the retinal pigment epithelium (RPE)/Bruch membrane. The majority of axial lengthening of the eye occurs within the first 3–6 months of life.
  - Newborn: 16 mm
  - 3 years: 22.5 mm
  - 13 to 18 years (adult length): 24 mm
- Length from lens to retina is 17 mm in adults.

2.2 MYOPIA

In myopia, the principle focus of light lies before reaching the retina. It can be defined as low ($<-3D$), moderate ($-3D$ to $-6D$) or high ($>-6D$). Myopia can be caused by:

- Axial myopia: Large eyes (axial length >24 mm). Most common cause.
- Index myopia: High refractive power as seen in conditions such as keratoconus or nuclear sclerotic cataract.

Methods that may be helpful in slowing myopic progression but there is no strong evidence for any strategy:

- Use of atropine (lower doses of atropine were more effective with fewer side effects than higher doses [1]) and pirenzepine drops.
- Outdoor activity: It is thought that too much near work may contribute in myopic progression (2).
- Bifocals and progressive lenses.

MANAGEMENT
- Spherical concave lenses (glasses or contact lenses).
- Keratorefractive surgery: Uses laser to reshape the cornea and so changing its refractive power. In myopia, the central corneal tissue is ablated, making the central cornea flatter. Common procedures used are photorefractive keratectomy (PRK), LASIK or LASEK.
  - *Caution*: Contact lens wearers should withhold wearing their lenses for at least 14 days for soft lenses and at least 1 month for rigid gas-permeable (RGP) lenses. Similarly, this precaution is used for hypermetropic surgery.

2.3 HYPERMETROPIA

In hypermetropia, the principle focus of light lies beyond the retina. It can be defined as low ($<+2D$), moderate ($+2D$ to $+5D$) or high ($>+5D$). Hypermetropia can be caused by:

- Small eyes (axial length <24 mm)
- Low refractive power: As seen in aphakic patients (absence of the lens) and patients with flat corneas

Associations of hypermetropia include esotropia, angle-closure glaucoma, retinoschisis, uveal effusion syndrome (nanophthalmos) and amblyopia in children.

MANAGEMENT

- Spherical convex lenses.
- Keratorefractive surgery: Procedures used are similar to those used in myopia; however, the peripheral corneal tissue is ablated in hypermetropia resulting in a steeper central cornea.

2.4 CONCEPTS RELATING TO MYOPIA AND HYPERMETROPIA

2.4.1 Spherical convex lenses

These are also called minus lenses, and they resemble two prisms placed base to base (Figure 2.1). They work by converging light and are used in managing hypermetropia by bringing the image formed behind the retina closer to land on the retina.

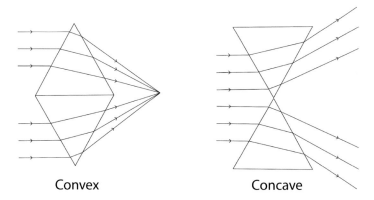

Convex   Concave

Figure 2.1 Convex versus concave lenses.

2.4.2 Spherical concave lenses

These are also called plus lenses and they resemble two prisms placed apex to apex (Figure 2.1). They work by diverging light and are used in managing myopia by bringing the image formed in front of the retina further to land on the retina.

2.4.3 Calculating the power lenses

The power of the lens is measured in diopters. It is equal to the reciprocal of the focal length (f) in metres:

$$\text{Power} = 1/f \tag{2.1}$$

SCENARIO

A hypermetropic patient is struggling to read at 33 cm. What power of convex lens is needed to aid his reading?

Answer:

- Power $= 1/f = 1/0.33 = 3D$.
- In hypermetropia, a plus lens is needed. Thus, the final answer is +3D.

2.5 ASTIGMATISM

Astigmatism occurs when the refractive power of the eye is not the same in all meridians (directions) due to a change in the shape of the lens or cornea's curvature, frequently described as 'rugby ball-shaped'. Patients usually are unable to distinguish letters such as 'o' and 'c'. Normal eyes can exhibit diurnal variations in corneal shape, flattest in the morning, as a result of changes in eyelid pressure and muscle tension (3).

TYPES OF ASTIGMATISM

- Regular astigmatism: The principle meridians, termed *steepest* and *flattest* meridians, are 90° from each other. Further classified as:
  - With-the-rule astigmatism: Occurs when the vertical meridian (90°) is the steepest. It is corrected with a plus cylinder lens between 60° and 120°.
  - Against-the-rule: Occurs when the horizontal meridian (180°) is the steepest. It is corrected with a plus cylinder lens between 150° and 30°.
  - Oblique: Occurs when the principle meridians are neither at 90° nor 180°. It is corrected with a plus cylinder lens between 31° and 50° and 121°–149°.
- Irregular astigmatism: Principle meridians are not perpendicular to each other. Occurs in conditions such as keratoconus or corneal ulcers.

MANAGEMENT OF ASTIGMATISM

- Soft toric lenses: Combination of spherical and cylindrical lenses.
- RGP contact lenses are usually used for irregular astigmatism.

2.6 CONCEPTS RELATING TO ASTIGMATISM

Cylindrical lenses are lenses that contain a cylinder in a single plane surface, and unlike spherical lenses, they focus the light into a line rather than a point. Hence, a spherical lens has the same power in all meridians, whereas a cylindrical lens has power in one meridian only.

2.6.1 Transposition

Transposition of prescription lenses/glasses refers to converting a minus cylindrical lens to a plus cylindrical lens and vice versa. This method, however, does not change the optical properties. This method is frequently used in toric lens prescriptions.

The steps of transposing:

- Step 1: Add the cylinder and sphere power; this becomes your new sphere power.
- Step 2: Change the sign of the cylinder.
- Step 3: Change the axis by 90°: If the axis is ≤90° then add 90°, but if it is >90° then subtract 90°.

SCENARIO

A patient has the following lens prescription: +3DS/−1DC at 90°. What is the transposition equivalent?

Answer: The first thing to understand is what the components mean:

- The +3DS is the power of the spherical component of the toric lens; in this case, we can tell it is a convex lens.
- The −1DC is the power of the cylindrical lens.
- The axis, 90°, describes the lens meridian that contains no cylinder power; in other words, it is perpendicular to the meridian that contains cylinder power.

Using the steps of transposing above, you will reach +2DS/+1DC at 180°. This is similar to saying +3DS/−1DC at 90°.

2.7 PRESBYOPIA

Presbyopia refers to an age-related loss of accommodative ability of the eye. It can be either due to an increase in lens size and hardness, or due to ciliary muscle dysfunction (4). Therefore, the lens cannot thicken or flatten properly, and accommodative power is lost. Accommodative power is 14D at the age of 8 years; presbyopia starts at about the age of 40 and the accommodative power is almost completely lost after the age of 60 (<1D).

2.8 CONCEPTS RELATING TO PRESBYOPIA

2.8.1 Calculating the amplitude of accommodation

- The amplitude of accommodation is the maximum increase in diopter power the eye can achieve through accommodation.
- The near point of the eye is the closest point where the image remains clear.
- To achieve comfortable vision, at least 1/3 of the amplitude of accommodation should be kept in reserve.

SCENARIO

A patient sees clearly at 33 cm but with any less the image becomes blurry. He wishes to see clearly at 25 cm. What power correction does he need?

- *Answer*: +2D correction.
- *Explanation*:
  - He sees clearly at 33 cm (near point). This means his amplitude of accommodation is +3D (Power = 1/f = 1/0.33).
  - To see comfortably he needs at least 1/3 of his accommodative amplitude in reserve. This means he can only use +2D (of his +3D power).
  - To be able to see clearly at 25 cm. He needs +4D power (Power = 1/f = 1/0.25). This means he needs an extra +2D power correction.

2.9 SQUINTS

Squints are broadly split into tropias and phorias. The conditions themselves are covered in Chapter 6, 'Strabismus'. In this section, we consider the role of prisms in the management of tropias.

2.9.1 Esotropia/exotropia

Esotropia is where the eye is deviated nasally and moves temporally on cover testing to fixate. Exotropia is where the eye is deviated temporally and moves nasally on cover testing to fixate. The angle of deviation can be measured objectively via prism cover testing.

When prescribing prisms, they should be placed for both eyes with the power of prisms split evenly between the two eyes. The base of the prism should point away from the deviation. For example, the base is pointed temporally in an esotropic eye and the apex nasally.

2.9.2 Hypertropia/hypotropia

Hypertropia is where the eye is deviated superiorly and moves inferiorly on cover testing to fixate. Hypotropia is where the eye is deviated inferiorly and moves superiorly on cover testing to fixate.

Again, the power of prisms should be split evenly between the two eyes. The base of the prism should be away from the deviation. Prisms should be pointing in opposite directions for both eyes. For example, for a right hypertropia, the right eye has the prism base down and the left eye has the prism base up.

2.10 CONCEPTS RELATING TO PRISMS

A prism is a transparent medium bound by two planes that are at an angle to each other. They do not focus light. They bend light (refraction) towards the base of the prism. To an observer, a virtual image is formed that is erect and displaced towards the apex (Figure 2.2).

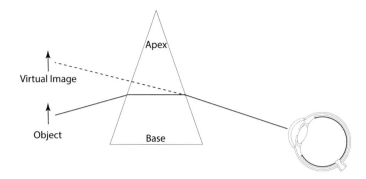

Figure 2.2 Image formed by prisms.

2.10.1 Refraction of light

Refraction follows Snell's law, which states that when light moves from one transparent medium of higher density to another of lower density (e.g. water to air), the light refracts. This concept applies to the eyes and is the basis for lens manufacturing.

2.10.2 Critical angle and total internal reflection

The angle of incidence is the angle the light travels as it hits the boundary of another medium. The angle of refraction is dependent on the angle of incidence and is the angle the light travels as it crosses the boundary.

When the angle of incidence increases, the angle of refraction gets closer to 90°. When the angle of refraction is equal to 90°, the angle of incidence is named the *critical angle*.

Total internal reflection occurs when the angle of incidence is greater than the critical angle; the light will not pass through the medium, that is, it is completely reflected. Optical instruments such as prisms and gonioscopy rely on this principle of total internal reflection.

2.10.3 Power of prism

One prism diopter (PD) produces a deviation of a light ray of 1 cm measured at 1 m from the prism. It can be calculated using one of two equations:

$$P = Fd \tag{2.2}$$

where P is the prism power (PD), F is the lens power (D) and d is the distance (cm) of the pupil from optical centre. Or

$$P = 2 \times \text{angle of deviation} \tag{2.3}$$

where the angle of deviation is measured in degrees (°).

SCENARIO 1

A patient has a 15° deviation esotropia of the right eye. What prism power and direction should be prescribed?

- *Answer:* 15PD base out (temporally) for both eyes.
- *Explanation:* P = 2 × angle of deviation = 30PD. Prisms should be split equally between the two eyes and the base should be away from the direction of squint.

SCENARIO 2

A patient has a right hypertropia and requires 30PD correction. What prism power and direction should be prescribed?

- *Answer:* 15PD base down right eye and 15PD base up left eye.
- *Explanation:* The power should be split evenly across the two eyes and the bases should be opposite directions.

SCENARIO 3

A patient complains of vertical diplopia. His glasses prescription is +2D (OD) and +1D (OS). His eyes are 5 mm down from the optical centre. What prism prescription should he have?

- *Answer:* 1PD base up right eye and 0.5PD base down left eye.
- *Explanation:* In hypertropia/hypotropia, the bases of the prisms should be in opposite directions.
  - OD: P = Fd = 2 × 0.5 = 1PD
  - OS: P = Fd = 1 × 0.5 = 0.5PD

2.11 MEASURING VISUAL ACUITY

2.11.1 Subjective measurements

1. SNELLEN CHART

   This is the most commonly used tool to subjectively assess visual acuity. The chart is placed 6 metres away from the patient (this represents the numerator). The denominator represents the distance at which an average person or eye can read. This means that a patient with 6/6 vision can read the letter at a distance of 6 metres of which an average person can read at 6 metres. Moreover, a 6/12 vision is where the patient can read a letter at 6 metres away that an average eye can read at 12 metres away.

   The Snellen chart starts with one letter at the top and as you read down the letters increase by one. Letter size is defined as the distance in metres that each letter subtends an angle of 5 minutes of arc.

2. DUOCHROME TEST

   This is a test that uses chromatic aberrations of the eye to refine the best vision sphere following optical correction. The test is comprised of black letters positioned on two backgrounds, red and green. As red is a longer wavelength than green, it will focus behind the retina, while green will focus in front of the retina.

The patient is asked to occlude one eye at a time and determine whether the black letters look clearer on the green or red backgrounds. If the patient doesn't see a difference, that means the circle of least confusion is on the retina and that is his perfect sphere correction. If the patient sees the black letters better on the red side, it means the focus is behind the retina (has a degree of hypermetropia), this is either because he has an under plus sphere or an over minus sphere. The opposite is true if the patient says green is better than red.

3. ISHIHARA CHART

This is a test used to screen for red-green colour vision defect. The test comprises of plates containing dots of various colours and sizes and other dots which form certain numbers that should be visible to a patient with normal colour vision.

4. LogMAR CHART

Due to limitations of the Snellen chart, a new chart was developed by Bailey and Lovie called the logarithm of minimum angle of resolution (LogMAR) chart (Figure 2.3). This chart is predominantly used for research purposes

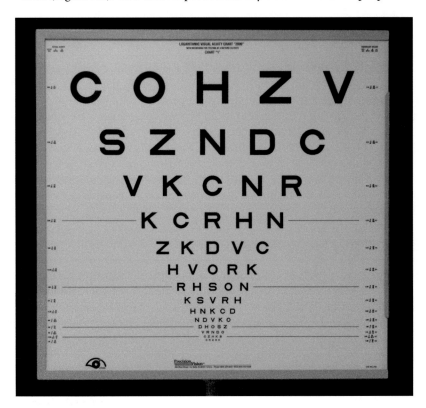

Figure 2.3 LogMAR chart.

due to it being more accurate. However, it is also used in clinical practice by some clinicians.

Key Features

- It has five letters on each row with equal spacing, ensuring the task is equivalent at each level and accounts for the crowding phenomenon (difficulty of recognizing letters when they are presented with other neighbouring letters. This occurs in amblyopia).
- The letter spacing is equal to one letter width.
- The row spacing is equal to the height of a letter from the row below.
- Each correct letter is worth 0.02 log units. Since there are five letters a line, a correct line is worth 0.1 log units.
- Patients are usually positioned 4 metres away. The scoring is from 1 to 0, so that each letter read correctly will result in subtraction of 0.02 from 1. In comparison with the Snellen chart, a 6/6 Snellen acuity is equal to 0 LogMAR and a 6/60 Snellen acuity is equal to 1 LogMAR.

2.11.2 Objective measurement

RETINOSCOPY

Retinoscopy is an objective method of measuring VA. It is useful in uncooperative patients.

Light from a retinoscope is shone into the patient's retina at a certain distance. The aim is to observe the patient's red reflex while adding plus/minus lenses until a complete red reflex is observed. In myopic patients, the direction of the reflex is against the direction of the light. In hypermetropic patients, the direction of reflex is with the direction of light.

Once the perfect reflex is observed, the examiner should subtract the dioptric equivalent of their working distance from the correcting lens. If the working distance is a 67 cm (2/3 m), then the examiner should subtract 1.5D (Power $= 1/f = 1/0.67$) from the lens power used to achieve perfect vision correction.

2.11.3 Visual acuity development

The visual acuity (VA) of children and adults differs. Cognitive function also differs, and hence different charts are used to assess patients of different ages and literacy. At birth, the vision is very poor, and infants are just able to fixate on objects or faces. By the age of 3 months, the infant is able to fixate and follow objects, and by the age of 5 months, they may develop full colour vision.

The average VA of different age groups is as follows:

- Newborn: 6/200–6/60
- 3 months: 6/90–6/60

- 6 months: 6/30
- 9 months: 6/24
- 1 to 2 years: 6/18–6/6

2.11.4 Testing visual acuity of different age groups

- Forced preferential looking charts (e.g. Keeler or Cardiff): Used for children less than 1 year of age.
- Cardiff cards: Used for children aged 6 months up to and including 2 years.
- Kay pictures: Children aged 2–3 years.
- Sheridan-Gardiner: Children aged 3–5 years.
- Snellen and LogMAR: Can be used for children over 4 years old and literate adults. The Keeler LogMAR or the illiterate E test (either Snellen or LogMAR) can be used for preschool children and illiterate adults.

2.12 OPTICS OF SLIT LAMPS

The slit lamp consists of two microscopes positioned at 13–14° from each other to provide a binocular view with stereopsis. There are also different types of illumination techniques which aid visualization of ocular structures:

- Direct (focal) illumination: Here the beam focusses on the part of the eye being examined. This is the most commonly used type and is appropriate in most situations.
- Diffuse illumination: This is where the illumination light is out of focus and diffusely illuminating the area being examined. Used for general examination of external eye structures.
- Retroillumination: Uses the light reflected from the iris to look for corneal opacities, or from the fundus to examine the red reflex, patency of iridotomies and lens opacities. Iris transillumination uses light reflected from the retina in an undilated pupil to view iris abnormalities, such as in pigment dispersion or pseudoexfoliation.
- Specular reflection: Best way to view corneal endothelium, for example, in Fuchs' corneal dystrophy.
- Sclerotic scatter: Light is directed at the limbus, which is in turn scattered through the cornea. Used to evaluate general corneal opacities.

2.13 OPTICS OF DIRECT OPHTHALMOSCOPY

A direct ophthalmoscope produces:

- An image with ×15 magnification and an area of about 2 disc diameters.
- An image that is virtual and erect.
- No stereoscopic vision.

2.14 OPTICS OF INDIRECT OPHTHALMOSCOPY

An indirect ophthalmoscope has a light attached to a headband and uses a handheld biconvex aspheric lens ranging from 15–40D in power. Generally, a 20D is routinely used. This produces an image that:

- Has a 2–5 times magnification. As the power increases, the magnification decreases; a 20D lens has about ×3 magnification, whereas a 30D lens has about ×2 magnification.
- Has a wide view of about 8 disc diameters.
- Is real and inverted vertically and horizontally.
- *Note:* The field of illumination is largest in cases of high myopia and smallest in hypermetropia.

REFERENCES

1. Chia A, Lu Q-S, Tan D. Five-year clinical trial on atropine for the treatment of myopia 2: Myopia control with atropine 0.01% eyedrops. *Ophthalmology.* 2016;123(2):391–9.
2. Rose KA, Morgan IG, Ip J, Kifley A, Huynh S, Smith W, Mitchell P. Outdoor activity reduces the prevalence of myopia in children. *Ophthalmology.* 2008;115(8):1279–85.
3. Read SA, Collins MJ, Carney LG. The diurnal variation of corneal topography and aberrations. *Cornea* .2005;24(6):678–87.
4. Glasser A, Croft MA, Kaufman PL. Aging of the human crystalline lens and presbyopia. *Int Ophthalmol Clin.* 2001;41(2):1–15.

3

Eyelids

OMAR KOULI, MOSTAFA KHALIL AND STEWART GILLAN

3.1 ANATOMY AND PHYSIOLOGY

The eyelid consists of (anterior to posterior):

1. Skin
2. Orbicularis oculi
3. Fibrous layer
4. Levator palpebrae superioris muscle
5. Müller muscle

3.1.1 Skin

The skin consists of epidermis, dermis and skin adnexa. The upper eyelid sits 2 mm inferior to the superior limbus (covering 1/6 of the cornea). The lower eyelid sits at the inferior limbus border.

SKIN ADNEXA

The adnexa lie deep in the dermis and includes the eyelashes and many types of glands:

- Eccrine glands: Sweat glands.
- Apocrine glands: Modified sweat glands (e.g. gland of Moll).
- Holocrine glands: Gland of Zeis, and meibomian glands. These glands synthesize/secrete lipids and oily substances.

SENSORY SUPPLY

- Lateral upper eyelid: Lacrimal nerve (CNV_1).
- Upper eyelid: Supraorbital and supratrochlear nerves (branches of frontal nerve of CNV_1).
- Medial canthal area: Infratrochlear nerve (branch of nasociliary nerve of CNV_1).
- Lower eyelid: Infraorbital nerve (CNV_2).

3.1.2 Orbicularis oculi

A striated muscle arranged in concentric bands that functions in closing the eye. It has four parts: palpebral, orbital, lacrimal and ciliary parts. Nerve supply is via temporal and zygomatic branches of CNVII.

3.1.3 Fibrous layer

Consists of tarsal plates and orbit septum (see Chapter 5). Tarsal plates provide structural support to the eyelid, and the upper tarsal plate is thicker than the lower tarsal plate.

3.1.4 Levator palpebrae superioris

A striated muscle responsible for eyelid retraction that originates at the lesser wing of the sphenoid to insert into the tarsal plate. Nerve supply is via the superior division of CNIII.

3.1.5 Müller muscle

A smooth muscle innervated by the sympathetic nervous system which contributes to eyelid retraction. Originates from the aponeurosis of the levator to insert into the tarsal plate.

3.1.6 Blinking reflex

The blinking reflex can be activated via different pathways depending on the stimulus:

- Corneal stimulus: CNV_1 (afferent), CNVII (efferent)
- Light stimulus: CNII (afferent), CNVII (efferent)
- Auditory stimulus: CNVIII (afferent), CNVII (efferent)

3.1.7 Bell's phenomenon

Bell's phenomenon is a physiological term referring to the upward and outward rotation of the globe on forced lid closure. This is particularly obvious in patients with CNVII palsy, as the lid remains open when patients are asked to close their eyes. This phenomenon is regarded as a defensive mechanism. However, it may be absent in about 10–15% of people.

3.2 CHALAZION

This is a sterile lipogranuloma that occurs due to obstruction of the meibomian glands and occasionally the gland of Zeis. It presents over several weeks as a painless round nodule in the eyelid (Figure 3.1). If infected, it may become red, swollen and painful. Associations include blepharitis and acne rosacea.

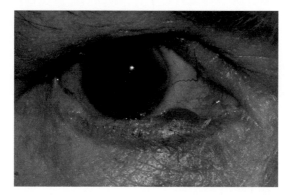

Figure 3.1 A chalazion.

Management is mainly with hot compresses twice daily and use of oral antibiotics if infected. Incision and curettage is also an option.

3.3 PORT WINE STAIN (NAEVUS FLAMMEUS)

A congenital capillary malformation of the dermis. They present as pink/purple well-demarcated patches that do not blanch on pressure and never cross the midline. Typically, they occur along the distribution of choroidal neovascularization (CNV). It may be associated with *Sturge-Weber syndrome.*

3.4 BASAL CELL CARCINOMA

Basal cell carcinoma (BCC) is the most common malignant eyelid tumour. They are slow growing and rarely metastasize.

HISTOPATHOLOGY

Clusters of darkly staining basaloid cells with peripheral palisading arrangement of nuclei.

FEATURES

- Centrally ulcerated pearly edged papules with associated telangiectasia (Figure 3.2)

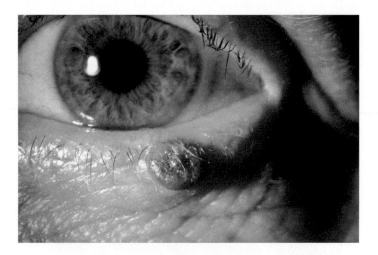

Figure 3.2 A basal cell carcinoma on the lower eyelid.

- Location (from most common to least common)
  - Eye: Lower lid > medial canthus > upper lid > lateral canthus
  - Lips: Upper lip > lower lip

MANAGEMENT

Mohs micrographic surgical excision (layered excision of the tumour to allow better total clearance).

3.5 SQUAMOUS CELL CARCINOMA

Squamous cell carcinoma (SCC) is less common than BCC. They are aggressive tumours and have the ability to metastasize to regional lymph nodes.

FEATURES

- Keratotic (e.g. scaly, crusty), ill-defined nodule that may ulcerate.
- Dome-shaped nodule with keratin-filled crater is typical in keratoacanthoma.

MANAGEMENT

Mohs surgery and radiotherapy.

3.6 SEBACEOUS GLAND CARCINOMA

This tumour arises from meibomian glands or, less commonly, glands of Zeis. On histopathology, foamy vacuolated lipid-containing cytoplasm with hyperchromatic nuclei are seen. They are more common in elderly females and appear as a yellow nodule in the upper eyelid which may be mistaken for a chalazion.

3.7 TRICHIASIS

- Misdirected growth of eyelash follicles, in which eyelashes grow towards the cornea or sclera (Figure 3.3).
- Most common causes: Herpes zoster ophthalmicus and blepharitis.

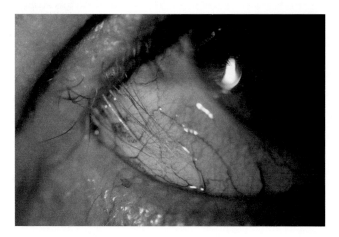

Figure 3.3 Trichiasis.

3.8 DISTICHIASIS

Refers to the formation of a posterior row of eyelashes. This may be congenital (AD inheritance) or acquired from chemical injury, Stevens-Johnson syndrome or ocular cicatricial pemphigoid.

3.9 BLEPHARITIS

Blepharitis is subdivided into anterior and posterior blepharitis.

- Anterior blepharitis: Inflammation of the skin around the base of the eyelashes and is divided into staphylococcal or seborrheic.
- Posterior blepharitis: Inflammation of the meibomian gland around the eyelid margins due to gland dysfunction. May be associated with ocular rosacea.

RISK FACTORS

- Dry eyes
- Seborrheic dermatitis
- Demodex folliculorum: Associated with ocular rosacea
- Long-term contact lens wear

CLINICAL FEATURES

- Symptoms: Bilateral and symmetric, dry, gritty, crusted and red eyes
- Signs:
  - Staphylococcus anterior blepharitis
    - Associated with atopic dermatitis
    - Lid hyperaemia and swelling
    - Hard scales and crusting of the bases of the lashes (Figure 3.4)
    - Tear film instability, dry eye syndrome and trichiasis may develop

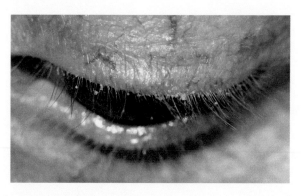

Figure 3.4 Scales and crusting in chronic staphylococcus anterior blepharitis.

  - Seborrheic anterior blepharitis
    - Associated with seborrheic dermatitis
    - Soft scales and oily lid margins
  - Posterior blepharitis
    - Associated with acne rosacea
    - Foamy and unstable tear film (due to abnormal meibomian gland secretion, leading to excess lipid in tear film)
    - Posterior lid margin hyperaemia and telangiectasia

TREATMENT

- Eyelid hygiene is the most important management.
- Antibiotics (e.g. tetracyclines, due to their ability to inhibit fatty acid oxidation and lipase production).
- Tea tree oil may be used for demodex infestation.

3.10 PTOSIS

Ptosis refers to the drooping of the upper eyelid. There are various causes, such as neurogenic (e.g. Horner syndrome, CNIII palsy), myogenic (e.g. myasthenia gravis, myotonic dystrophy), involutional (age-related) or congenital (due to failure of development of the levator muscle).

3.10.1 Marcus Gunn jaw-winking syndrome

Occurs in 5% of patients with congenital ptosis. It presents as a ptotic lid that retracts when the ipsilateral pterygoid muscle is stimulated (e.g. chewing).

3.11 PSEUDOPTOSIS

Includes dermatochalasis, blepharochalasis, microphthalmus and phthisis bulbi (atrophic, non-functioning eye that occurs as a result of severe ocular disease).

3.11.1 Dermatochalasis

Excessive skin of the upper eyelid leading to sagging, classically described as lateral hooding. This condition occurs in the elderly.

3.11.2 Blepharochalasis

This bilateral condition results from abnormal elastic eyelids causing recurrent episodes of painless oedema of the upper eyelids. This leads to stretching and atrophy of the skin and subsequent skin folds and ptosis.

3.12 FLOPPY EYELID SYNDROME

Typically occurs in middle-aged obese men with obstructive sleep apnoea. The upper eyelid is extremely lax, which may lead to papillary conjunctivitis and keratopathy.

3.13 LID RETRACTION

Lid retraction can occur in both upper and lower eyelids. It may be physiological (e.g. in shallow orbits or large eyes) or secondary to underlying disease.

CAUSES

- Graves ophthalmopathy
- Parinaud syndrome (*Collier sign*)
- Third nerve misdirection
- Marcus Gunn jaw-winking syndrome
- Progressive supranuclear palsy
- Down syndrome
- Congenital hydrocephalus (setting-sun appearance: bilateral downward deviation of the globes with upper lid retraction)

3.14 LID COLOBOMA

Incomplete development of the eyelid due to the failure of lid fold fusion. It can occur in either the upper or lower eyelids.

3.14.1 Upper eyelid

Forms at the junction of the middle and inner thirds of the upper eyelid. Can be associated with Goldenhar syndrome.

3.14.1.1 GOLDENHAR SYNDROME

A sporadic condition characterized by upper lid coloboma, microphthalmia, optic disc coloboma, maxillary and mandibular hypoplasia, and limbal dermoids (smooth yellow subconjunctival mass, typically at the inferotemporal limbus with hair protrusion). May be associated with Duane retraction syndrome.

3.14.2 Lower eyelid

Forms at the junction of the middle and outer thirds of the lower eyelid. Can be associated with Treacher Collins syndrome.

3.15 HORDEOLUM (STYE)

External hordeolum is an infection of the glands of Zeis or Moll. Internal hordeolum is an infection of the meibomian gland. It is usually due to a staphylococcal infection and presents as a painful, erythematous swelling of the eyelid. Management includes hot compresses, topical antibiotics and eyelid hygiene.

4

Lacrimal system and dry eyes

OMAR KOULI, MOSTAFA KHALIL AND STEWART GILLAN

4.1 ANATOMY AND PHYSIOLOGY

4.1.1 Tear film

Composed of three layers with different composition and functions (Table 4.1).

4.1.2 Lacrimal system

Pathway: Lacrimal gland → puncta → canaliculi → Lacrimal sac → nasolacrimal duct → inferior nasal meatus.

LACRIMAL GLAND

- The lacrimal gland is a tubule-alveolar gland consisting of acini and ducts. Acini are responsible for the production of watery secretions.
- The lacrimal gland consists of two parts:
  - Orbital part: Lies in the frontal bone.
  - Palpebral part: Located superolaterally in the eyelids, inferior to the levator palpebrae muscle.
- Function: Forms the aqueous layer of the tear film.

Table 4.1 Tear film composition

Layer	Lipid (superficial)	Aqueous	Mucous (deep)
Source	Meibomian glands	Lacrimal gland (reflex secretion) and accessory lacrimal glands (basal secretion)	Conjunctival goblet cells
Function	Prevent aqueous layer evaporation	Antibacterial activity, washing out debris and supplying cornea with nutrients	Aids in spreading tears and stabilizing the tear film
Thickness	0.1 μm	7.0 μm	0.2 μm

- Blood supply: Lacrimal artery, a branch of the ophthalmic artery.
- Nerve supply
  - Sensory: Lacrimal nerve (CNV_1).
  - Parasympathetic secretomotor: CNVII. Pathway: preganglionic parasympathetic fibres originate from the superior salivatory nucleus in the pons and travel with the greater petrosal nerve (a branch of the CNVII) to synapse at the pterygopalatine ganglion. Postganglionic fibres then joins the lacrimal branch of CNV1 to supply the lacrimal gland.
- Lacrimal reflex: CNV_1 (afferent) and CNVII (efferent).

ACCESSORY LACRIMAL GLANDS

These glands are histologically similar to the lacrimal gland. They sustain the basal secretory level of the aqueous layer of the tear film.

- Krause glands: Situated adjacent to the conjunctival fornix. They are more numerous in the upper eyelid.
- Wolfring glands: Situated in the upper border of the tarsal plate. Although fewer in number, they are larger than Krause glands.

PUNCTA

A small, round opening located medially at the posterior edge of the upper and lower lid margins at the junction of the lid's ciliated and non-ciliated parts.

CANALICULI

The superior and inferior canaliculi are comprised of:

- A vertical part, the ampulla (2 mm long).
- A second horizontal part, about 8 mm long, after the vertical part.

The superior and inferior canaliculi then join together at the common canaliculus. The junction of the lacrimal sac and common canaliculus contains the Rosenmuller valve, which is important in preventing tear reflux.

LACRIMAL SAC

Situated in the lacrimal fossa, which is formed by the lacrimal bone and frontal process of the maxilla.

NASOLACRIMAL DUCT

- Continuation of the lacrimal sac.
- Opens into the inferior meatus in the nose.
- The opening contains a fold of mucous called the valve of Hasner. This valve functions to prevent air entering the nasolacrimal system during nose blowing.

4.2 ACQUIRED OBSTRUCTION

The main presenting complaint is epiphora. Causes and treatment include the following.

PUNCTAL STENOSIS

- Causes: Idiopathic or chronic blepharitis.
- Treatment: Punctoplasty.

NASOLACRIMAL OBSTRUCTION

- Causes: Idiopathic, trauma, surgery or tumours.
- Treatment: Dacryocystorhinostomy (anastomosis of lacrimal sac with mucosa of middle meatus).

4.3 CONGENITAL NASOLACRIMAL DUCT OBSTRUCTION

Newborn infants may present with congenital nasolacrimal obstruction. Around 90% of cases resolve within the first 12 months of life. The obstruction is typically at the valve of Hasner.

FEATURES

- Epiphora
- Mucopurulent discharge on pressure over lacrimal sac

TREATMENT

- First line: Observation and massaging of the lacrimal sac for the first 12 months of life.
- Second line: Nasolacrimal duct probing.
- Third line: Nasolacrimal duct stent insertion, balloon dilatation or dacryocystorhinostomy.

4.4 CANALICULITIS

This is an infection of the canaliculi most commonly due to *Actinomyces israelii*. Usually presents unilaterally with epiphora, red eye and discharge on pressure over the canaliculus. Management is with topical antibiotics.

4.5 DACRYOADENITIS

An idiopathic lacrimal gland inflammation. Tear stasis is the main risk factor. Secondary causes include viral infections (e.g. mumps). Bilateral dacryoadenitis should raise suspicion of sarcoidosis. Persistence or presence of paraesthesia should raise concern of carcinoma.

FEATURES

- Painful, tender, erythematous and swollen lacrimal gland (superolateral upper eyelid).
- Disturbed tear production.
- S-shaped ptosis of the upper eyelid.
- Downward and inward displacement of the globe.

4.6 DACRYOCYSTITIS

Infection of the lacrimal sac due to an obstruction in the nasolacrimal duct. Most commonly due to *Staphylococcus aureus, S. epidermidis* (in adults), *Streptococcus pneumoniae* or *Haemophilus influenzae* (in children).

FEATURES AND MANAGEMENT

- Acute
  - Erythematous, tender swelling over the lacrimal sac with associated epiphora.
  - Treat with warm compresses, systemic antibiotics and dacryocystorhinostomy after the acute phase has completely resolved to reduce the risk of recurrence.
- Chronic
  - Epiphora and recurrent unilateral conjunctivitis.
  - Treat with dacryocystorhinostomy.

4.7 PLEOMORPHIC ADENOMA OF THE LACRIMAL GLAND

Most common lacrimal gland tumour, occurring in middle-aged patients. Benign, but can transform into malignant.

- Histopathology: Epithelial and mesenchymal components.
- Features: Progressive, painless enlargement of the upper eyelid with inferonasal dystopia.
- Investigation: CT scan.
- Treatment: Surgical excision.

4.8 LACRIMAL GLAND CARCINOMA

A rare, malignant tumour of the lacrimal gland.

- Histopathology: The main type is adenoid cystic carcinoma, which exhibits a cribriform or 'Swiss cheese' growth pattern. Other types include pleomorphic adenocarcinoma and mucoepidermoid carcinoma.
- Features: Rapidly growing and painful lacrimal gland mass, inferonasal dystopia, optic disc swelling, choroidal folds and may cause perineural invasion (spreading of a cancer around a nerve causing neurological deficits).
- Management: Biopsy, orbital exenteration (surgical removal of the globe and surrounding tissue), radical orbitectomy and/or radiotherapy.

4.9 SJÖGREN SYNDROME

An autoimmune condition in which the salivary and lacrimal glands become infiltrated with lymphocytes and the acini are progressively destroyed.

FEATURES

- Triad: Xerostomia, keratoconjunctivitis sicca and parotid gland enlargement.
- Posterior blepharitis is commonly present.
- Corneal punctate epithelial erosions (stains with fluorescein).
- Strands of filaments containing mucus or debris (stains with rose bengal).

INVESTIGATIONS

- Anti-Ro and anti-La antibodies.
- Reduced tear film breakup time.
- Schirmer test: Determines whether the eye produces enough tears to keep it moist.
- Ocular staining: Showing interpalpebral staining of cornea and conjunctiva, rather than a superior or inferior stain pattern seen in superior limbic keratoconjunctivitis or exposure keratopathy, respectively.

MANAGEMENT OF DRY EYE

- First line: Ocular lubricants and artificial tears: includes hypromellose (lowest viscosity), carbomer and paraffins (highest viscosity).
- Second line: Topical corticosteroids and/or oral pilocarpine (increases lacrimal gland secretion).
- Third line: Punctal occlusion or low-water content bandage contact lenses (e.g. silicone hydrogel).

4.10 XEROPHTHALMIA

Xerophthalmia is caused by severe vitamin A deficiency, which is a major cause of childhood blindness in Africa.

FEATURES

- Nyctalopia
- Xerosis: Severe conjunctival dryness and keratinization
- Bitot's spots: Triangular keratinized buildup on the conjunctiva
- Punctate corneal epithelial erosions
- Keratomalacia in severe cases

MANAGEMENT

Vitamin A supplementation and topical lubrication.

5

Orbit

MOSTAFA KHALIL, OMAR KOULI AND RIZWAN MALIK

5.1 ANATOMY

5.1.1 Bony orbit

The orbit is a pyramidal-shaped space with the apex situated posteriorly and the base anteriorly. It is madeup of seven bones which are grouped as follows:

- Roof: Frontal bone and lesser wing of the sphenoid.
- Lateral wall: Zygomatic bone and greater wing of the sphenoid.
- Floor: Zygomatic, maxillary and palatine bones.
- Medial wall: Maxillary, lacrimal, sphenoid and ethmoid bones. The *lamina papyracea* is a paper-thin plate which covers the ethmoidal cells and forms a part of the medial wall. It can act as a route of entry for infection from the ethmoid sinus.

5.1.2 Orbital openings

1. Optic foramen: Located within the lesser wing of the sphenoid. It transmits the optic nerve and ophthalmic artery into the middle cranial fossa.
2. Superior orbital fissure (SOF): Located between the greater and lesser wings of the sphenoid. It is divided into two parts:
   - Superior part: Contains the superior ophthalmic vein, the lacrimal nerve (CNV_1), the frontal nerve (CNV_1) and the CNIV.
     - *Note*: The frontal nerve branches into the supraorbital and supratrochlear nerves. The supraorbital nerve leaves the orbit via the supraorbital notch.
   - Inferior part: Contains CNIII, the nasociliary nerve (CNV_1) and CNVI.
3. Inferior orbital fissure: Located between the maxilla and the greater wing of the sphenoid bone. It contains the infraorbital nerve (CNV_2), the zygomatic nerve (CNV_2) and the inferior ophthalmic vein.
   - *Note*: The infraorbital nerve exits the orbit via the infraorbital foramen.

Surrounding the optic canal and the inferior part of the SOF is the common tendinous ring (annulus of Zinn). The annulus of Zinn is a fibrous tissue marking the origin of the four recti muscles. Through it run the CNII, CNIII, CNVI and the nasociliary nerve.

Note: Retrobulbar anaesthetic block affects the nerves inside the common tendinous ring.

5.1.3 Orbital septum

- The orbital septum is located anterior to the orbit and extends from the orbit rims to the eyelid.
- It is a membranous sheet that forms the fibrous part of the eyelids.
- It is an important landmark as it marks the border between the periorbital (preseptal) and orbital (postseptal) regions.

5.2 THYROID EYE DISEASE

Thyroid eye disease (TED) is the most common cause of unilateral and bilateral axial proptosis in adults. It is an idiopathic autoimmune disorder consisting of an *active inflammatory phase* (months-years) in which the eyes are red and painful, followed by an *inactive fibrotic phase* that involves extraocular muscles (EOM) and connective tissues. Peak incidence is at 30–50 years.

It is usually associated with hyperthyroidism but may be also associated with hypothyroidism or euthyroid patients.

RISK FACTORS

- Smoking
- Females
- HLA-DR3 and HLA-B8

PATHOPHYSIOLOGY

- Sympathetic overstimulation of the Müller muscle due to high levels of thyroid hormones causing eyelid retraction.
- Fibroblastic deposition of glycosaminoglycans into the EOM producing oedema and eventual fibrosis of EOM. This leads to:
  - Impaired movement of EOM (restrictive myopathy).
  - Exophthalmos which exposes the cornea causing dryness, irritation and exposure keratitis.
  - Lid retraction due to fibrosis of levator palpebrae.
  - Increased pressure on the optic nerve causing optic neuropathy.
  - Impaired venous drainage leading to conjunctival and periorbital oedema and conjunctival injection.

CLINICAL FEATURES

- Unilateral/bilateral axial proptosis, redness, chemosis and ocular irritation.
- Lid retraction (Dalrymple sign).
- Lid lag on downgaze (Von Graefe sign).
- 'Staring' appearance (Kocher sign).
- Restrictive myopathy: EOM is usually affected in the following order: inferior rectus (IR), medial rectus (MR), superior rectus (SR), levator palpebrae, lateral rectus (LR).
- Choroidal folds (rare).

INVESTIGATIONS

- Thyroid function tests.
- Imaging
  - CT or MRI are indicated if orbital decompression is planned, to help confirm an equivocal diagnosis or if there is asymmetry on exophthalmometry.
  - Shows thickening of EOM bellies (most commonly IR and MR) with characteristic tendon sparing.
- Visual field testing is indicated, especially if optic neuropathy is suspected.

MANAGEMENT

The management of TED is directed according to the severity of the condition. TED can be classified, according to the European Group on Graves' Orbitopathy (EUGOGO) (1), into *severe sight-threatening* (optic neuropathy), *moderate-severe* (exophthalmos $\geq$3 mm, lid retraction $\geq$2 mm and/or diplopia) and *mild* disease. The management of TED according to EUGOGO is as follows.

General measures

- Smoking cessation.
- Achieve euthyroid status.

Mild disease

- Watchful waiting.
- Ocular lubricants during day and overnight to avoid dryness and ulceration of the cornea.

- Topical ciclosporin to reduce ocular irritation.
- Overnight lid taping for mild exposure keratopathy.
- Selenium supplements can improve the course of TED (2).

Moderate-severe disease

- IV methylprednisolone ± oral prednisolone: Bisphosphonates should be considered in patients receiving steroid therapy due to risk of osteoporosis. It is important to check liver function in patients receiving high doses of IV steroids.
- Orbital radiotherapy: Can be used in combination with steroids or when steroids are contraindicated in patients with active TED complaining of diplopia or restricted eye movements. Orbital irradiation can increase risk of retinopathy in diabetic and hypertensive patients.
- Surgery
  - Surgery is indicated after inflammatory phase subsides (i.e. in the inactive phase), in cases of optic neuropathy, significant proptosis, persistent diplopia or severe lid retraction.
  - The following order is recommended if surgery is indicated:
    – Orbital decompression
    – Strabismus surgery
    – Eyelid surgery

COMPLICATIONS AND ASSOCIATIONS

- Dysthyroid optic neuropathy: Causes severe sight-threatening TED, suspect if there are changes in colour vision or VA with presence of optic disc swelling and relative afferent pupillary defect (RAPD). Treatment is with IV steroids and orbital decompression (if unresponsive to IV steroids).
- Exposure keratopathy: Manage with lubricants, surgery (e.g. tarsorrhaphy) or botulinum toxin injections.
- Superior limbic keratoconjunctivitis: A common association with TED.

5.3 ORBITAL CELLULITIS AND PRESEPTAL CELLULITIS

Preseptal cellulitis and orbital cellulitis refer to the infection of soft tissues anterior and posterior to the orbital septum, respectively (Table 5.1).

5.4 ORBITAL MUCORMYCOSIS

Presentation is similar to orbital cellulitis but with more gradual onset and occurs in immunocompromised patients or patients with diabetic ketoacidosis. It is caused by the fungal family *Mucoraceae*. Symptoms include orbital swelling and signs of orbital cellulitis. Characteristically, necrotic *black eschars* over the nasal turbinates or palate can form.

Table 5.1 Orbital cellulitis versus preseptal cellulitis

Condition	Orbital cellulitis	Preseptal cellulitis
Background	Infection of the soft tissues of the eye socket behind the orbital septum	Infection isolated anterior to the orbital septum
Aetiology	Spread of infection from paranasal sinuses most commonly ethmoidal sinus	Direct inoculation from eyelid trauma
Common organisms	*Streptococcus pneumoniae, Staphylococcus aureus* and *Haemophilus influenzae*	*Staphylococcus aureus, Streptococcus pyogenes* and *Streptococcus pneumoniae*
Features	• Children are most commonly affected • Acute onset of swelling of orbital tissue, chemosis and limited eye movement and proptosis • Fever, tenderness and restricted eye movement • RAPD, decreased colour vision, dVA and diplopia may occur	• Patient presents with eyelid oedema and erythema with associated low-grade fever • Important distinctions from orbital cellulitis include normal eye movement, normal VA and colour saturation, absence of proptosis and absent of RAPD
Investigations	CT scan	CT scan if doubtful diagnosis
Management	Admit for IV antibiotics (e.g. ceftriaxone + flucloxacillin + metronidazole)	Oral antibiotics (e.g. co-amoxiclav)
Complications	Orbital abscess Cavernous sinus thrombosis Brain abscess and meningitis Optic neuropathy	Can progress to orbital cellulitis

5.5 RHABDOMYOSARCOMA

Rhabdomyosarcoma is considered the most common primary orbital malignancy in children. The mean age of onset is 8 years (3). The most common affected areas are the genitourinary system and the head and neck (including orbit).

HISTOPATHOLOGY

This tumour has the ability to differentiate into striated muscle from undifferentiated mesenchymal cells. Embryonal is the most common subtype and is characterized by elongated spindle-shaped cells ('strap cells') (3).

CLINICAL FEATURES
- Rapidly progressive unilateral proptosis.
- Most common location in the orbit is superonasal.
- Diplopia may occur.

INVESTIGATION
- MRI or CT: Shows a circumscribed mass ± bone erosion.
- Biopsy.

5.6 NEUROBLASTOMA

This is the most common extracranial solid tumour in children and is derived from the neural crest cell of the sympathetic nervous system. It most commonly occurs in the adrenal medulla secreting catecholamines but can also involve the head, neck, chest abdomen or spine. It usually metastasises to the orbit.

- Histology: Homer-Wright rosettes.
- Clinical features: Child with unilateral/bilateral proptosis and periorbital ecchymosis (racoon eyes). Differential for basal skull fracture.
- Association: Opsomyoclonus, a rare neurological syndrome characterized by conjugate jerky eye movements (dancing eyes) and cerebellar ataxia (dancing feet).

5.7 LYMPHANGIOMA

Rare vascular hamartomatous tumours which may form blood-filled 'chocolate' cysts. They present in childhood and depend on whether the lesion is anterior or posterior.

ANTERIOR LYMPHANGIOMA

Soft bluish mass superonasally on eyelid or conjunctiva which are exacerbated by Valsalva manoeuvre.

POSTERIOR LYMPHANGIOMA

Insidious growth may lead to proptosis. Presentation can be with painful proptosis due to spontaneous haemorrhage.

5.8 OPTIC NERVE GLIOMA VERSUS OPTIC NERVE SHEATH MENINGIOMA

Tumours affecting the optic nerve can arise from either the glial tissue, such as optic nerve glioma, or from the meninges, such as optic nerve sheath meningioma (Table 5.2).

5.9 CAROTID-CAVERNOUS FISTULA: DIRECT VERSUS INDIRECT

Carotid-cavernous fistula (CCF) refers to the development of an arteriovenous connection between the cavernous sinus (venous) and the carotids (arterial). The connections can be either direct or indirect (Table 5.3).

5.10 CAVERNOUS HAEMANGIOMA

This is the most common benign hamartoma of the orbit in adults. It is a low-flow arteriovenous malformation. It is commonly located within the muscle cone,

Table 5.2 Optic nerve glioma versus optic nerve sheath meningioma

Condition	Optic nerve glioma	Optic nerve sheath meningioma
Background	Slow-growing benign tumour which typically affects children	Slow-growing benign tumour which typically affects middle-aged females
Associations	Neurofibromatosis 1	Neurofibromatosis 2
Clinical features	Gradual painless, monocular proptosis, visual loss and RAPD Optic nerve head can be initially swollen but then becomes atrophic	Pathogenomic triad of progressive, painless and unilateral visual loss + optic atrophy + optociliary shunt vessels; proptosis may also occur
Investigations	CT: Fusiform enlargement of the optic nerve	CT: Thickening of the optic nerve sheath ('tram-track' sign) and osteoblastic changes

Table 5.3 Direct versus indirect CCF

Condition	Direct CCF	Indirect CCF
Background	A high-flow arteriovenous fistula or communication between the cavernous sinus and internal carotid artery directly	A low-flow arteriovenous fistula or communication between meningeal branches of the internal/external carotids and the cavernous sinus
Aetiology	Usually due to trauma (can be spontaneous)	Usually spontaneous and most commonly in hypertensive elderly women

Features	• Acute onset following head injury
	• Triad
	  • Pulsatile proptosis with associated bruit
	  • Conjunctival chemosis
	  • Whooshing sound in head
	• Ophthalmoplegia (due to cranial nerve damage)
	• Raised IOP
	• Papilloedema
	• Visual loss
		• Gradual onset of redness and irritation of the eyes
		• Raised IOP
		• Moderate venous dilatation with later tortuosity of retinal vasculature
		• Corkscrew epibulbar vessels
		• Mild proptosis

Investigations	• CT/MRI: Dilatation of the superior ophthalmic vein • Definitive diagnosis: MRA, CRA or angiography	Same as Direct CCF
Management	Transarterial repair of the artery (embolization)	• Spontaneous resolution in about half of the cases • Monitor IOP and VA
Complications	• Immediate visual loss due to optic nerve damage at the onset of head injury • Delayed visual loss can be due to open-angle glaucoma (most common cause of visual loss)	N/A

lateral to the optic nerve. It is more common in middle-aged females and typically unilateral in presentation.

CLINICAL FEATURES

- Slowly progressive axial proptosis. Most notable during pregnancy.
- Induced hypermetropia due to globe indentation.
- Optic nerve compression may occur, leading to decreased VA (dVA).
- Extraocular muscle restriction leading to diplopia.

INVESTIGATIONS

- USS shows a well-defined intraconal lesion with increased reflectivity.
- CT or MRI can show a well-circumscribed lesion, typically intraconally.

MANAGEMENT

- Surgical excision if vision affected.

5.11 CAPILLARY HAEMANGIOMA

A type of hamartoma; the most common benign orbital tumour of infancy. These are high-flow endothelial neoplasms which undergo rapid growth due to vascular endothelial growth factor soon after birth.

- May be superficial ('strawberry naevi') or deep (posterior to orbital septum).
- More common in boys.
- Rapid growth in early infancy (2 months–1 year) with spontaneous regression by 7 years of age.

CLINICAL FEATURES

- Bright red unilateral lesion on upper eyelid which blanch with pressure or enlarge when the child cries (Valsalva).
- Ptosis due to its location in the upper lid.
- Deep lesions, however, are dark blue/purple in colour and can cause axial proptosis.

MANAGEMENT

- Observation: Most resolve spontaneously.
- If risk of amblyopia, cosmetic reasons or anisometropic astigmatism
  - Propranolol
  - Corticosteroid injections or systemic steroids
  - Surgical excision

5.12 CAVERNOUS SINUS THROMBOSIS

Cavernous sinus thrombosis refers to a clot formation within the sinus and is mainly due to a spreading infection from the paranasal sinuses, ear or pre-existing orbital cellulitis.

CLINICAL FEATURES

- Rapid-onset headache, nausea, vomiting, chemosis and dVA.
- Unilateral or bilateral proptosis.
- Diplopia due to CNIII, CNIV or CNVI compression. CNVI is first to be affected, as it lies freely within the cavernous sinus, causing a lateral gaze palsy.

INVESTIGATIONS

- MRI and MRI venography to confirm diagnosis.

MANAGEMENT

- Intravenous antibiotics, steroids and/or low-molecular-weight heparin.
- Surgical drainage.

COMPLICATIONS

- Meningitis
- Septic emboli
- CNS deficits

REFERENCES

1. Luigi B, Baldeschi L, Dickinson A et al. Consensus statement of the European Group on Graves' Orbitopathy (EUGOGO) on management of GO. *Eur J Endocrinol.* 2008;158(3):273–85.
2. Marcocci C, Kahaly GJ, Krassas GE et al. Selenium and the course of mild Graves' orbitopathy. *N Engl J Med.* 2011;364(20):1920–31.
3. Karcioglu ZA, Hadjistilianou D, Rozans M, DeFrancesco S. Orbital rhabdomyosarcoma. *Cancer Control* 2004;11(5):328–33.

6

Strabismus

AHMED HASSANE, RIZWAN MALIK AND OBAID KOUSHA

6.1 ANATOMY AND PHYSIOLOGY

6.1.1 Extraocular muscles

Six extraocular muscles, four recti and two oblique, are responsible for moving the eye. The medial rectus has the closest insertion to the limbus (5.5 mm) while the superior rectus has the furthest insertion from the limbus (7.7 mm). Table 6.1 summarizes the muscle origins, innervation and functions.

6.1.2 Principles of extraocular muscle movement

ANTAGONIST-AGONIST MUSCLES

Muscles in the same eye that move the eye in different directions. For example, left MR (adduction) and left LR (abduction).

SYNERGIST MUSCLES

Muscles in the same eye that move that eye in the same direction. For example, right IR (depression) and right SO (depression).

Table 6.1 Extraocular muscles and their functions

Muscle	Origin	Innervation	Primary function	Secondary function
Superior rectus	Annulus of Zinn	CNIII	Elevation	Intorsion and adduction
Inferior rectus	Annulus of Zinn	CNIII	Depression	Extorsion and adduction
Medial rectus	Annulus of Zinn	CNIII	Adduction	N/A
Lateral rectus	Annulus of Zinn	CNVI	Abduction	N/A
Superior oblique (SO)	Lesser wing of sphenoid	CNIV	Intorsion	Abduction and depression
Inferior oblique (IO)	Orbital floor	CNIII	Extorsion	Abduction and elevation

YOLK MUSCLES

Muscles, one in each eye, that cause the two eyes to move in the same direction (Figure 6.1). For example, the right LR and the left MR are responsible for right gaze, and hence they are termed yolk muscles.

Ocular Movement

Figure 6.1 The ocular movements of both eyes.

HERING'S LAW

States that yolk muscles involved in a particular direction of gaze receive equal and simultaneous flow of innervations. For example, contraction of the MR is accompanied by equal contraction of the contralateral LR.

SHERRINGTON'S LAW

States that an increase in innervation of a muscle is accompanied by a decrease in innervation of its antagonist. For example, when the left LR contracts, the left MR relaxes.

6.2 IMPORTANT DEFINITIONS

6.2.1 Amblyopia

Amblyopia is characterized by a reduction in VA in the early years of life (<8 years of age) due to a developmental failure of the visual pathway between the eye and the visual cortex in the occipital lobe. It is usually unilateral and is caused by abnormal stimulation due to various aetiologies.

- Aetiologies: Strabismus, refractive error and stimulus deprivation (e.g. cataract).
- Management
  - Treat underlying cause.
  - Occlusion therapy: The good eye is patched to allow visual connections between the amblyopic eye and the brain to develop properly.
  - Pharmacologic penalisation of the good eye using atropine. (*Note*: Atropine may cause photophobia and reverse amblyopia.)

6.2.2 Binocular single vision

Ability to fuse images from both eyes to produce a single image. Characteristics of binocular vision are as follows.

- Simultaneous perception: An image formed simultaneously on each retina.
- Fusion
  - Sensory fusion: The ability to unite the two images from each retina to form a single image.
  - Motor fusion: The ability to align the eyes to maintain sensory fusion. Motor fusion occurs via version (conjugate movements) and vergence (disconjugate movements) in order to achieve binocular vision.
- Stereopsis: Perception of depth.

6.2.2.1 TESTS FOR BINOCULAR STATUS

- Simultaneous perception and fusion
  - Worth 4-dot test, Bagolini glasses and synoptophore.
- Motor fusion
  - Base-out or base-in prism bar or Risley prism tests. Applying a base-out prism moves the image to the temporal retina so the eye has to converge to achieve binocular single vision. The opposite is true for a base-in prism.
- Stereopsis
  - Titmus, Lang, TNO, Frisby and synoptophore.

6.2.3 Heterophoria

Deviation of the eye that is hidden by fusion and revealed when fusion is broken, for example, with an alternating cover test.

- Esophoria: Inward deviation of the eye
- Exophoria: Outward deviation of the eye

6.2.4 Heterotropia

Abnormal alignment of the eye, also known as a manifest squint. Can be tested using the cover test.

- Esotropia: Convergent squint
- Exotropia: Divergent squint

6.2.5 Accommodative convergence to accommodation (AC/A) ratio

In the normal eye, one diopter of accommodation is accompanied by 3–5 PD of accommodative convergence. The AC/A ratio might be abnormal in different types of strabismus.

6.3 ESOTROPIA

The most common form of childhood squint in the UK. Esotropia can be caused by a variety of conditions including nerve palsies, thyroid eye disease, trauma among others. It can be classified into accomodative or non accomodative.

6.3.1 Accommodative esotropia

Accommodative esotropia is due to refractive errors or convergence excess. It usually presents in patients between 1 and 5 years old and is associated with hypermetropia. Several subtypes exist.

FULLY ACCOMMODATIVE ESOTROPIA

Esotropia that resolves with correction of hypermetropia. Normal AC/A ratio. Management includes a full cycloplegic hypermetropic correction.

PARTIALLY ACCOMMODATIVE ESOTROPIA

Esotropia that partially resolves with correction of hypermetropia. Normal AC/A ratio. Management includes a full cycloplegic hypermetropic correction and treatment of amblyopia.

CONVERGENCE EXCESS ESOTROPIA

Esotropia for near vision only due to high convergence. High AC/A ratio. Management includes bifocal glasses or surgery (e.g. bilateral MR recession).

6.3.2 Non-accommodative esotropia

Infantile esotropia develops within the first 6 months of life and is the most common esotropia. Other types of non-accommodative esotropias exist and usually present after the first 6 months of life.

- Infantile esotropia
  - Large-angle (>30PD) deviation
  - Cross-fixation (carries low risk of amblyopia)
  - Latent horizontal nystagmus
- Near versus distance esotropia
  - Distance: Esophoria for near vision and esotropia for distance
  - Near: Esotropia for near only but with normal AC/A ratio

6.4 EXOTROPIA

Exotropia can be classified into constant or intermittent exotropia. Unlike esotropia, exotropia is associated with myopia.

6.4.1 Intermittent exotropia

This is the most common type of exotropia and can be split into *distance* and *near* exotropia. Distance exotropia can be further divided into *true* and *simulated distance* exotropia. Treatment is with myopic correction, orthoptic exercises or surgery (e.g. unilateral or bilateral LR recession).

DISTANCE EXOTROPIA

In true distance exotropia, there is an exotropia made worse looking at a distance with normal AC/A ratio.

In simulated distance exotropia, there is a larger exotropia for distance with high AC/A ratio; however, the near exotropia is increased when looking through a +3D lens or after occlusion of the normal eye.

NEAR EXOTROPIA

Defined as a worse exotropia for near vision, it is common in young myopic adults or teenagers.

6.4.2 Constant exotropia

A constant large-angle exotropia, typically occurring within the first 6 months of life. It is usually associated with neurological anomalies. Management is surgical with bilateral LR recession and MR resection.

6.5 MICROTROPIA

A small angle squint <10PD (5°), most commonly an esotropia associated with anisometropia. Patients have subnormal binocular single vision with sensory and motor fusion and reduced stereopsis. It is subclassified into microtropia with identity (no manifest deviation on cover test but deviation can occur on 4PD test) or microtropia without identity (manifest deviation on cover test).

Table 6.2 Duane retraction syndrome types (Huber classification)

Type	Features
I (most common)	Esotropia with limited abduction
II	Exotropia with limited adduction
III	Esotropia with limited abduction and adduction

Source: Huber, A. *Br J Ophthalmol.* 1974;58(3):293.

6.6 DUANE RETRACTION SYNDROME

This rare condition arises due to innervation of the LR muscle by CNIII rather than CNVI with associated CNVI nucleus hypoplasia. This causes characteristic retraction of the globe on adduction. Associated with deafness or Goldenhar syndrome. Three types exist (Table 6.2).

6.7 BROWN SYNDROME

This unilateral syndrome is caused by mechanical restriction of the SO tendon at the trochlea. It can be congenital or arise post-trauma/surgery. The most common feature is limited elevation in adduction or on upgaze with an associated click sensation.

6.8 PRINCIPLES OF STRABISMUS SURGERY

RESECTION VERSUS RECESSION

Resection is the process of shortening the muscle (strengthening procedure). Recession is the process of loosening the muscle by moving it away from its insertion (weakening procedure).

For example, in constant exotropia, bilateral LR recession (loosening) and MR resection (strengthening) corrects the eye misalignment.

OTHER STRENGTHENING PROCEDURES

Tucking is the procedure used to augment the SO muscle. Indication is for congenital fourth nerve palsy.

Advancement involves bringing the muscle closer to the limbus. This is done to a previously recessed EOM.

OTHER WEAKENING PROCEDURES

Disinsertion is primarily used for a highly active IO. It separates the tendon at its insertion, making it weaker.

REFERENCE

1. Huber A. Electrophysiology of the retraction syndromes. *Br J Ophthalmol.* 1974;58(3):293.

7

Neuro-ophthalmology

OMAR KOULI AND OBAID KOUSHA

7.1 ANATOMY

7.1.1 Optic nerve

CNII is formed by the convergence of retinal ganglion cell axons. The nasal axons of CNII correspond to the temporal visual field, while the temporal axons correspond to the nasal visual field. CNII has four parts:

1. Intraocular (shortest; 1 mm): Exits posteriorly via the lamina cribrosa (scleral opening).
2. Intraorbital (longest; 25 mm): Has myelinated covering. Ends at the optic foramen.

3. Intracanalicular: Where the optic nerve exits the orbit through the optic canal to enter the middle cranial fossa.
4. Intracranial: Ends at the optic chiasm.

CNII BLOOD SUPPLY

- Intraocular: Short posterior ciliary artery.
- Intraorbital to intracranial: Pial vessels of ophthalmic artery.

7.1.2 Optic chiasm

The chiasm is located anterior to the hypothalamus and usually directly superior to the pituitary gland. Within the chiasm, axons representing the temporal retina continue ipsilaterally. Axons representing the nasal retina decussate at the chiasm to the contralateral optic tract.

Interestingly, inferonasal axons turn anteriorly within the chiasm to join the contralateral CNII (*Wilbrand's knee*) before continuing back into the optic tract. This explains why anterior chiasmal lesions tend to cause junctional scotomas: ipsilateral optic neuropathy with contralateral superotemporal defects.

A few photosensitive retinal ganglion cell axons connect with the suprachiasmatic nucleus of the hypothalamus. This is important for the body's circadian rhythm.

7.1.3 Optic tract

The optic tracts connect the optic chiasm with the lateral geniculate nuclei (LGN). The optic tract conveys signals from the contralateral nasal retina and the ipsilateral temporal retina.

7.1.4 Optic radiations and occipital cortex

The optic radiations connect the LGN to the occipital lobe. Superior optic radiations, representing the inferior visual field quadrants, pass through the parietal lobe and terminate at the primary visual cortex (also known as V1 or Brodmann area 17) in the occipital lobe, superior to the calcarine sulcus (cuneus gyrus). The inferior optic radiations (Meyer's loop), representing the superior visual field quadrants, pass through the temporal lobe and terminate at the primary visual cortex, inferior to the calcarine sulcus (lingual gyrus). The macula is represented posteriorly just lateral to the tip of the calcarine sulcus.

7.1.5 Oculomotor nerve

The oculomotor nucleus is located in the dorsal midbrain at the level of the superior colliculus. Motor functions:

- Ipsilateral innervation to IO, IR and MR.
- Contralateral innervation to SR.
- Bilateral innervation to levator muscle.

PATHWAY

CNIII exits the brainstem through the interpeduncular fossa, passing between the posterior cerebral artery and superior cerebellar artery. Along its path, it travels near the uncus of the temporal lobe, making it vulnerable for compression in cases of uncal herniations. It then travels through the lateral wall of the cavernous sinus superior to CNIV and bifurcates into a superior and inferior branch at the anterior aspect of the sinus.

It enters the orbit through the SOF within the annulus of Zinn. The superior branch innervates the SR and the levator muscle, while the inferior branch innervates the MR, IR and IO.

CNIII is accompanied by parasympathetic fibres originating from the Edinger-Westphal nuclei, located in the midbrain dorsal to oculomotor nuclei, which innervates the sphincter papillae and ciliary body muscles.

7.1.6 Pupillary light reflex

The pupillary light reflex consists of the CNII (afferent limb), the interconnecting neurons in the midbrain and CNIII (efferent limb).

PATHWAY

The fibres involved in the pupillary pathway originate from the retinal ganglion cells. Those fibres exit the optic tract before reaching the LGN and enter the midbrain to synapse on the ipsilateral pretectal nucleus. The pretectal nuclei project bilateral fibres to the contralateral and ipsilateral Edinger-Westphal nuclei.

Preganglionic parasympathetic fibres from Edinger-Westphal travel along with CNIII and then exit the inferior branch of CNIII to synapse on the ciliary ganglion. From the ciliary ganglion, postganglionic parasympathetic fibres are carried via the short ciliary nerves to innervate the ciliary body muscle and sphincter pupillae.

7.1.7 Accommodation reflex

Accommodation is the adaptation of the eye when focusing on a near object. It works by:

1. Increasing lens curvature: The ciliary body muscles contract via parasympathetics from Edinger-Westphal, leading to relaxation of the lens zonules.
2. Pupil constriction: Activation of the sphincter pupillae via parasympathetics form Edinger-Westphal.
3. Eye convergence: Contraction of medial recti via CNIII.

7.1.8 Trochlear nerve

The trochlear nuclei are located in the midbrain at the level of the inferior colliculus. Each trochlear nucleus innervates the contralateral SO muscle. CNIV passes through the lateral wall of the cavernous sinus inferior to CNIII and enters the SOF above the common tendinous ring. CNIV characteristics include:

- Only cranial nerve to exit dorsally from the brainstem.
- Smallest cranial nerve in number of axons.
- Longest unprotected intracranial course.

7.1.9 Abducens nerve

The abducens nucleus is located in the pontine tegmentum ventral to the fourth ventricle. The nucleus is located near the paramedian pontine reticular formation (PPRF) and surrounded by looping fibres of CNVII. CNVI exits the brainstem at the pontomedullary junction and crosses over the petrous apex of the temporal bone through an osteofibrous channel, called Dorello's canal. It is at the Dorello's canal where CNVI is susceptible to stretching in cases of increased intracranial pressure. CNVI then travels *through* the cavernous sinus, lateral to the internal carotid. It then enters the orbit via the SOF, through the tendinous ring, to innervate the LR muscle.

7.1.10 Pathway for pupillary dilatation

The sympathetic nervous system is responsible for pupillary dilatation and contraction of Müller muscle.

PATHWAY

1. First-order neurons: Start at the posterolateral hypothalamus and synapse at the intermediolateral cell column between C8 to T2 (ciliospinal centre of Budge).
2. Second-order preganglionic neurons: Leave centre of Budge, travel over the lung apex and synapse at the superior cervical ganglion at the carotid bifurcation. This is where sudomotor fibres exit to course with the external carotid and supply the sweat glands of the face.
3. Third-order postganglionic neurons: Travel around the internal carotid artery to finally innervate the dilator pupillae via long ciliary nerves (branches of the nasociliary nerve).

7.1.11 Supranuclear eye movements

The eye movements are under voluntary or reflex control. The voluntary movements are initiated in the frontal eye field (FEF), Brodmann area 8, in the frontal lobe. The reflex movements are coordinated via the occipital cortex and superior colliculus in response to a visual stimulus.

Supranuclear motor control consists of three types of movements:

1. Saccadic eye movements
2. Smooth pursuit movements
3. Vestibulo-ocular movements

7.1.11.1 SACCADES

Saccades are fast eye movements which involve the rapid fixation of a desired object onto the fovea with abrupt change of point of fixation when switching from one object to the next. Saccades can have an angular speed of 600°/s, lasting around 30–100 milliseconds after a latency (time it takes to initiate) of approximately 200 milliseconds (1).

Voluntary horizontal saccadic eye movements are initiated by the FEF. Activation of the right FEF will result in the eyes looking to the left, and vice versa. Projections from FEF go directly, or via the superior colliculus, to the contralateral PPRF, which lies ventral to the abducens nucleus in the brainstem. The PPRF activates the ipsilateral abducens nucleus and sends impulses through the medial longitudinal fasciculus (MLF) to activate the contralateral oculomotor nucleus.

Vertical saccades are controlled via the rostral interstitial nucleus of the MLF (riMLF).

7.1.11.2 SMOOTH PURSUIT

This refers to slow movements of the eye designed to keep a moving stimulus fixed at the fovea. They have a latency of about 100 milliseconds, and a much slower velocity than saccades. They are initiated from parieto-occipital areas (2).

7.1.11.3 VESTIBULO-OCULAR MOVEMENTS

These eye movements stabilize the eye relative to head movements. When moving the head, with eyes fixed on an object, sensory information of the semicircular canals results in the movement of the eyes in the opposite direction to the head movement. This occurs via projections from the vestibular nuclei to cranial nerves and PPRF.

For example, if the head rotates rightward then the activity of the right vestibular nucleus increases whereas the left vestibular nucleus activity decreases. This causes the contraction of the ipsilateral MR and contralateral LR muscles and the relaxation of the contralateral MR and ipsilateral LR muscles.

7.2 OPTIC NEUROPATHY

Optic neuropathy refers to damage of the optic nerve. Optic atrophy occurs as a result of longstanding damage to the optic nerve. The common signs of optic nerve dysfunction are:

1. Decreased visual acuity (dVA)
2. Dyschromatopsia
3. Visual field defects: Central scotomas, arcuate or altitudinal defects
4. Diminished contrast sensitivity
5. Absolute or relative afferent pupillary defect (RAPD)

The causes are listed below under their respective headings.

7.2.1 Optic neuritis

Refers to the inflammation of CNII. It has three types:

1. Retrobulbar neuritis
   a. The optic nerve behind the globe is affected.
   b. The optic nerve head is not involved, giving rise to a normal-looking optic disc on funduscopy.
   c. More common in adults.
2. Papillitis
   a. Hyperaemia and oedematous optic disc with associated peripapillary flame-shaped haemorrhage.
   b. The optic nerve head is affected.
   c. More common in children, typically in post-viral infections.
3. Neuroretinitis
   a. Papillitis with involvement of the retina.
   b. Occurs in cat scratch disease and Lyme disease.

7.2.1.1 DEMYELINATING OPTIC NEURITIS

Acute demyelinating optic neuritis is the most common form of optic neuritis. It can occur in isolation or with conditions such as multiple sclerosis (MS) or neuromyelitis optica (Devic disease).

7.2.1.1.1 Multiple sclerosis

MS is an autoimmune inflammatory disorder characterized by demyelination of the CNS. It has a female predominance and mainly presents in the third or fourth decades of life. MS is also more common in countries further away from the equator.

Systemic features

- Paraesthesia.
- Muscle cramping and weakness.
- Bladder, bowel and sexual dysfunction.
- Cerebellar dysfunction: Tremor + dysarthria + ataxia (Charcot's triad).
- Lhermitte sign: Electrical shock on neck flexion.
- Uhthoff phenomenon: Symptoms worsen when body temperature increases (e.g. hot shower).

Ophthalmic features

- Retrobulbar optic neuritis: Acute onset of unilateral retrobulbar pain exacerbated by eye movements, dVA, central scotoma, dyschromatopsia and RAPD. This is followed by a spontaneous resolution after a few months (3).
- Internuclear ophthalmoplegia.
- Nystagmus.

Investigations

- MRI: Demyelinating plaques disseminated in space and time.
- Lumbar puncture: Oligoclonal bands in CSF.

Management

Intravenous methylprednisolone for 3 days followed by oral prednisolone for 11 days. This regimen resulted in a faster recovery and significant improvement in contrast sensitivity, colour vision and visual field compared to the oral prednisolone and placebo groups. However, methylprednisolone had only a slightly better but nonsignificant outcome in VA (3).

7.2.1.1.2 Neuromyelitis optica

A demyelinating disorder characterised by severe retrobulbar optic neuritis and transverse myelitis in three or more vertebral columns causing muscle weakness, increased tone and spasms. IgG antibodies against astrocytic aquaporin-4 (AQP4) can be found.

7.2.1.2 NEURORETINITIS

Inflammation of the optic nerve with oedema spreading from the optic nerve head along the papillomacular bundle to reach the macula. Formation of exudates around macula gives a 'macular star' appearance. It is mainly caused by cat-scratch disease:

- Organism: *Bartonella henselae* (Gram-negative rod).
- Transmission: Cat scratch or bite.
- Features
  - Fever and lymphadenopathy
  - Neuroretinitis: Unilateral, painless decrease in VA, papilitis, mild optic nerve dysfunction and star pattern of macular exudates
  - Uveitis
  - Granulomatous conjunctivitis

7.2.2 Anterior ischaemic optic neuropathy

Anterior ischaemic optic neuropathy (AION) occurs due to damage to the optic nerve as a result of ischaemia. It can cause optic neuropathy in the elderly due to occlusion of the short posterior ciliary artery. It can be split into non-arteritic and arteritic (Table 7.1).

7.2.3 Leber hereditary optic neuropathy

A mitochondrial inherited disease caused by ganglion cell degeneration. Mitochondrial DNA mutation occurs at the 11,778 (most common, worst

Table 7.1 Non-arteritic AION versus arteritic AION

	Non-arteritic AION	Arteritic AION
Aetiology	Hypertension, diabetes, sleep apnoea or a physiologically small or absent cup (structural crowding of the optic nerve head)	Most commonly due to GCA
Vision loss	Sudden Painless Unilateral VA usually >6/60 Visual field defect: Often inferior or superior altitudinal defects	Sudden Painful Unilateral with high risk to fellow eye if untreated Severe visual loss with VA <6/60
Disc findings	Usually segmental hyperaemic disc swelling with peripapillary splinter haemorrhages	'Chalky-white' diffuse swollen disc (Figure 7.1)
Associated symptoms	N/A	Scalp tenderness, headache and jaw claudication
Investigations	Blood pressure, blood sugar, examination of optic disc and exclude GCA FA: Delayed optic disc filling	ESR, CRP and temporal artery biopsy (specific but sensitivity can be low due to 'skip lesions') FA: Delayed choroidal and optic disc filling
Treatment	Treat underlying cause	High-dose IV methylprednisolone followed by oral prednisolone

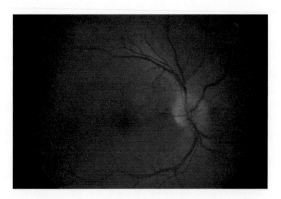

Figure 7.1 A 'chalky-white' oedematous disc in arteritic AION.

prognosis) or 14,484 (good prognosis). It mainly presents in young males aged 10–30 years. No effective treatment is available.

FEATURES

- Unilateral initially with bilateral ocular involvement over weeks to months.
- Painless visual loss.
- Central or centrocaecal scotomas.
- Triad of disc 'pseudo-oedema', peripapillary telangiectasia and tortuosity of the medium-sized retinal arterioles (Figure 7.2).
- Optic atrophy occurs in late disease.

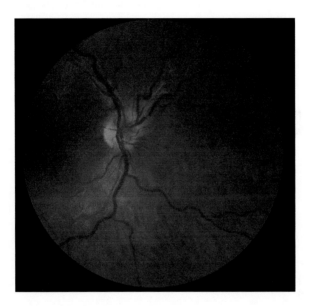

Figure 7.2 The classical triad of Leber hereditary optic neuropathy.

INVESTIGATION

- Family history and genetic testing.
- Optical coherence tomography (OCT): Can show optic nerve oedema (early) or atrophy (late).

7.2.4 Nutritional optic neuropathy

Also known as tobacco-alcohol amblyopia. It can be caused by vitamin B, copper and folic acid deficiencies, medications (e.g. ethambutol, amiodarone or sildenafil) and other toxic causes (smoking and alcohol).

FEATURES

- Gradual, progressive and painless bilateral dVA and centrocaecal scotomas.
- Dyschromatopsia.

7.2.5 Papilloedema

Bilateral optic disc swelling secondary to raised intracranial pressure (ICP). Causes of increased ICP include tumours, haemorrhages, hydrocephalus and idiopathic intracranial hypertension (a diagnosis of exclusion, typically occurs in young, obese females).

FEATURES OF INCREASED ICP

- Headache (worse in the morning) with nausea and/or vomiting.
- Pulsatile tinnitus.
- Unilateral or bilateral transient visual loss with a duration of seconds.
- Enlarged blind spot.
- Diplopia due to CNVI palsy (less common).
- Hypertension + bradycardia + bradypnea (Cushing reflex).
- Optic disc signs
  - Hyperaemia and blurred margins of optic disc (early)
  - Swelling and elevation of the whole optic disc with peripapillary haemorrhages (late) (Figure 7.3)

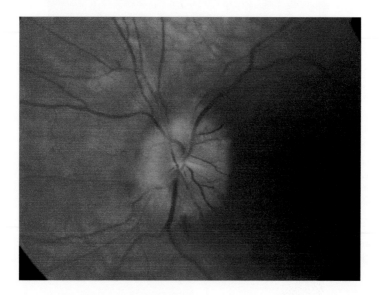

Figure 7.3 An established papilloedema.

7.2.6 Congenital optic disc anomalies

TILTED DISCS

- Bilateral, small optic discs tilted inferonasally.
- Associated with high myopia.
- Superotemporal field defects are common.

MORNING GLORY ANOMALY

- Unilateral and causes severe dVA.
- Characterized by a *funnel-shaped excavation* of the optic disc and surrounding retinal tissue. Characteristically, the retinal vessels emerge from the periphery of the optic nerve head rather than from the centre.
- Associated with retinal detachment.

OPTIC DISC PIT

- Characterized by a greyish oval depression in the optic nerve head, usually located temporally.
- Complications: Exudative retinal detachment.

OPTIC DISC COLOBOMA

- Occurs due to defect in embryonic fissure closing.
- Can be sporadic or associated with Goldenhar syndrome, microphthalmos, CHARGE syndrome and many others.
- Glistening white bowl-shaped excavation of the disc (inferior part predominantly affected) causing superior field defects and dVA.

OPTIC DISC DRUSEN

- Collection of mucoproteins and mucopolysaccharides that progressively calcify in the optic disc. They present as yellow or white bodies on the optic disc.
- Commonly bilateral.
- Varying degrees of blurring/visual loss.
- Associations: Retinitis pigmentosa and angioid streaks.

OPTIC NERVE HYPOPLASIA

Caused due to underdevelopment of the optic nerve. Patients often present with varying degrees of visual loss and a double-ring sign (Figure 7.4). Risk factors include genetic diseases and maternal use of recreational drugs, smoking and alcohol.

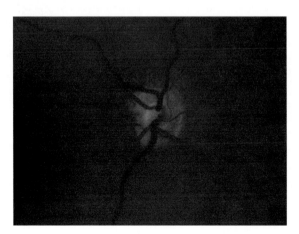

Figure 7.4 A hypoplastic optic nerve with a double-ring sign.

7.3 PUPILS

7.3.1 Physiological anisocoria

Anisocoria refers to the presence of asymmetrical pupillary size between the two eyes. It can be physiological or pathological. The normal pupil size is between 2–4 mm in light conditions and 4–8 mm in the dark (4).

Physiological anisocoria can be present in up to 20% of the population (5). The anisocoria is usually less than 1–1.5 mm in diameter and is unchanged in light and dark environments.

7.3.2 Horner syndrome

Caused by a lesion to the sympathetic pathway. Characterized by:

- Ptosis: Mild eyelid drooping due to Müller muscle dysfunction.
- Miosis: Due to dysfunction of the dilator pupillae. The pupil reacts to light and near stimuli.
- Ipsilateral facial anhidrosis: Not present in third-order neuron lesions.
- The affected iris in congenital Horner syndrome has a lighter colour.

CAUSES

- First order: Lateral medullary syndrome and syringomyelia.
- Second order: Pancoast tumour and neck trauma.
- Third order: Internal carotid dissection (painful), cluster headache and cavernous sinus lesions.

INVESTIGATIONS

- Topical apraclonidine (0.5% or 1%)
  - Used to confirm a Horner's pupil.
  - Apraclonidine is an alpha-2 and alpha-1 adrenergic agonist.
  - Causes pupillary dilation in the Horner's pupil due to denervation supersensitivity.
- Topical cocaine (4%)
  - Used to confirm a Horner's pupil.
  - Cocaine blocks the reuptake of noradrenaline.
  - Causes a pupillary dilation of the normal pupil more than the Horner's pupil.
- Topical hydroxyamphetamine (1%)
  - Used to differentiate a preganglionic from a postganglionic Horner's pupils.
  - Hydroxyamphetamine releases norepinephrine from normal postganglionic adrenergic nerve endings, causing pupillary dilation.
  - Failure of dilation if the lesion is postganglionic (third order); however, first- and second-order neuron lesions will dilate.
- CT or MRI: If tumours or carotid dissection/aneurysm are suspected.

7.3.3 Adie's pupil

A unilateral condition characterized by loss of postganglionic parasympathetic innervation to the iris sphincter and ciliary muscle.

FEATURES

- A large pupil with poor response to light but intense pupillary response (miosis) to near stimuli with slow re-dilation (light-near dissociation: pupil reaction to a near stimulus is greater than its reaction from a light stimulus).
- Holmes-Adie syndrome: Associated diminished deep tendon reflex of lower limbs.

INVESTIGATIONS

- Slit lamp: Vermiform movements of pupillary borders.
- Pharmacological: 0.1% (low dose) of topical pilocarpine into both eyes causes constriction of the affected pupil due to denervation hypersensitivity.

7.3.4 Argyll Robertson pupil

Characterized by bilateral, irregular small pupils. Both pupils do not react to light; however, they constrict normally on accommodation (*light-near dissociation*). The most common cause is diabetes; it was previously neurosyphilis.

7.4 CRANIAL NERVES

7.4.1 Optic nerve lesions

The visual field defects differ depending on the location of the lesion along the optic pathway (Figure 7.5).

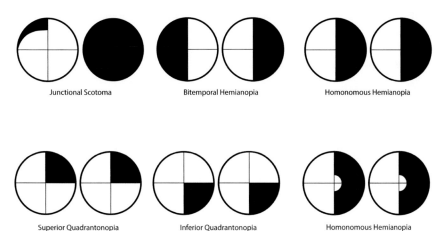

Figure 7.5 The visual field defects of the optic pathway.

CHIASMATIC

- Large pituitary adenomas
  - Bitemporal superior quadrantanopia which progress to *bitemporal hemianopia.*
- Craniopharyngioma
  - Bitemporal inferior quadrantanopia which can progress to *bitemporal hemianopia.*
  - Causes growth failure, delayed puberty, headaches, diabetes insipidus, obesity and hypothyroidism in children.
- Tuberculum sellae meningioma
  - Can affect the anterior angle of chiasm causing a junctional scotoma.
- Aneurysms
  - A large anterior communicating artery aneurysm may cause bitemporal hemianopia.
  - Bilateral internal carotid aneurysms may cause *binasal hemianopia* as they affect the temporal portions of the chiasm.

OPTIC TRACT

- Contralateral incongruous (asymmetrical) homonymous hemianopia.

OPTIC RADIATIONS

- Temporal radiations: Contralateral incongruous superior homonymous quadrantanopia 'pie in sky'.
- Parietal radiations: Contralateral incongruous inferior homonymous quadrantanopia 'pie in floor'.
- Main radiations: Contralateral incongruous homonymous hemianopia.

OCCIPITAL CORTEX

- Occlusion of the calcarine artery of the posterior cerebral artery: Contralateral congruous homonymous hemianopia with macular sparing.
- Damage to the tip of the occipital cortex due to systemic hypoperfusion or following an injury to the back of the head: Congruous homonymous hemianopic central scotoma.

7.4.2 CNIII lesions

AETIOLOGY

Causes of CNIII palsy can be split into medical or surgical problems.

Medical problems such as diabetes and hypertension are the most common causes; they affect the blood supply to the nerve. However, they are usually pupil-sparing, as pupillomotor fibres are located superficially within the nerve and are supplied by pial blood vessels (which are not affected in these conditions).

Surgical problems, however, are pupil involved, as the pupillomotor fibres are damaged or compressed. Surgical causes include posterior communicating artery aneurysm, trauma and uncal herniation.

FEATURES

- Ptosis.
- Abduction and depression of the eye in primary position ('down and out') with ophthalmoplegia (only abduction of the eye is fully normal).
- Dilated pupil and accommodation abnormalities.

7.4.2.1 VASCULAR SYNDROMES OF CNIII PALSIES

Weber syndrome

- CNIII palsy
- Contralateral hemiparesis (damage to the cerebral peduncle)

Benedikt syndrome

- CNIII palsy
- Contralateral hemiataxia and hemitremor (damage to the red nucleus)

Nothangel syndrome

- CNIII palsy
- Ipsilateral cerebellar ataxia (damage to the superior cerebellar peduncle)

Claude syndrome

- Benedikt + Nothangel

7.4.3 CNIV lesions

AETIOLOGY

Common causes include congenital CNIV palsy, closed head trauma and microvascular ischaemia.

FEATURES

- Vertical diplopia: Worse on walking downstairs or looking down.
- Hypertropia: The affected eye is higher than the contralateral eye. It is made worse on tilting the head to the ipsilateral shoulder.
- Depression of the eye is limited: Most noted on adduction.
- Compensatory head posture to avoid diplopia: Patients tend to develop a contralateral head tilt and face turn.
- Bilateral CNIV palsies can present with compensatory depressed chin posture and crossed hypertropia.

EXAMINATION

The Park-Bielschowsky three-step test can be used to identify a superior oblique palsy. Note that the complete three steps may not always be all positive (6). The three steps are:

1. Identify hypermetropic eye in primary position.
2. Eyes are examined in left and right gazes. Hypertropia increases on opposite gaze in CNIV palsy (worse on opposite gaze [WOOG]).

3. With the patient fixating at a target ahead, assess hypertropia on right and left head tilts. Hypertropia gets better on contralateral head tilt in CNIV palsy (better on opposite tilt [BOOT]).

7.4.4 CNVI lesions

AETIOLOGY
- Microvascular ischaemia (most common).
- Other causes: Trauma, idiopathic and ICP.

FEATURES
- Horizontal double vision: Worse on looking at distant targets.
- Esotropia in primary position.
- Abduction is limited.

7.4.4.1 SIXTH NERVE SYNDROMES
Foville syndrome
- Lesion to the inferior medial pons
- CNVI palsy
- Ipsilateral facial numbness (CNV)
- Ipsilateral facial paralysis (CNVII)
- Loss of taste sensation to the anterior two-thirds of the tongue
- Horner syndrome

Millard-Gublar syndrome
- Lesion to the ventral pons
- CNVI palsy
- Contralateral hemiplegia due to damage to the corticospinal tract
- Ipsilateral CNVII palsy

Gradenigo syndrome
- Causes: Otitis media, mastoiditis or petrositis
- Periorbital pain unilaterally (CNV)
- Diplopia (CNVI palsy)
- Otorrhoea

7.5 GAZE ABNORMALITIES

7.5.1 Internuclear ophthalmoplegia

- Lesion to the MLF, commonly caused by demyelination or stroke.
- Defective adduction of the eye ipsilateral to the lesion and abducting nystagmus of the contralateral eye.
- Patients may complain of horizontal diplopia.

7.5.2 One-and-a-half syndrome

- Lesion to the PPRF and MLF on the same side, commonly caused by a stroke.
- The only movement left is the abduction of the contralateral eye.

7.5.3 Parinaud syndrome

- Lesion to the dorsal midbrain.
- Causes: Pinealoma or aqueductal stenosis in children and vascular problems in adults.
- Supranuclear upgaze palsy.
- Lid retraction (Collier sign).
- Convergence-retraction nystagmus.
- Large pupil with light-near dissociation (not reactive to light but constrict on accommodation).

7.5.4 Progressive supranuclear palsy

A neurodegenerative progressive disorder characterized by vertical gaze palsy, slowing of vertical saccades, postural instability and parkinsonism.

7.6 NYSTAGMUS

Nystagmus is an involuntary rapid and repetitive oscillation of the eye which can be physiological or pathological. There is a risk of amblyopia in young patients with nystagmus, so it is important to correct refractive error and treat the underlying cause.

7.6.1 Physiological

- End-point nystagmus: Nystagmus at extreme gaze.
- Optokinetic nystagmus: Nystagmus due to fast-moving repetitive objects.

7.6.2 Pathological

7.6.2.1 CONGENITAL NYSTAGMUS

- The nystagmus is horizontal, pendular or jerky and disappears during sleep. It often has a null point – a position of gaze where nystagmus is minimal.
- Common causes include sensory deprivation (e.g. bilateral cataracts), optic nerve hypoplasia or foveal hypoplasia (e.g. albinism).

7.6.2.2 ACQUIRED NYSTAGMUS

Latent nystagmus

- Horizontal and jerky nystagmus, but only becomes present on monocular occlusion (direction is away from the covered eye).
- Most commonly associated with infantile esotropia.

Convergence-retraction nystagmus

- Co-contraction of horizontal muscles on attempted upgaze causing the globe to retract.
- The medial rectus is the most powerful EOM. This causes eye convergence.
- Caused by dorsal midbrain lesions (e.g. Parinaud syndrome).

Upbeat nystagmus

Downward drifting of the eye followed by a fast upward corrective saccade or beat. Caused mainly due to medulla lesions.

Downbeat nystagmus

Upward drifting of the eye followed by a fast downward corrective saccade or beat. Caused mainly due to lesions at the craniocervical junction such as Arnold-Chiari malformations.

Peripheral vestibular nystagmus

A conjugate horizontal and jerky nystagmus that occurs due to a vestibular lesion (e.g. labyrinthitis). There is a slow drifting of the eyes towards the side of the lesion followed by a fast corrective saccade in the other direction.

7.7 MYASTHENIA GRAVIS

An autoimmune disease affecting the post-synaptic nicotinic acetylcholine receptors (AChR) at neuromuscular junctions, leading to muscle fatigability. It typically presents in the third decade of life and has a female predominance.

It affects voluntary muscles, and smaller muscles are affected first. Ocular involvement is commonly the presenting feature.

FEATURES

- Ptosis: Bilateral (can be unilateral initially), worse at end of the day or after prolonged upgaze.
- Cogan lid twitch: A brief upshoot of the lid elicited by making patient look downwards then upwards.
- Diplopia.
- Ophthalmoplegia.
- Fatigability and weakness of muscles of facial expression and proximal limb muscles.
- Respiratory depression.

INVESTIGATIONS

- Ice test: Ptosis improves after applying ice for 2 minutes.
- Antibodies: Anti-AChR antibody and anti-muscle-specific kinase (MUSK) antibody.
- Repetitive nerve stimulation (decrement of muscle action potential amplitudes).
- CT thorax: Can reveal a thymoma.

MANAGEMENT

- Acetylcholinesterase inhibitors (e.g. pyridostigmine), steroids and immunomodulators.
- Thymectomy if thymoma is present.

7.8 MYOTONIC DYSTROPHY

Myotonic dystrophy is characterised by abnormal muscular relaxation and muscle wasting. It is an AD condition due to tri-nucleotide repeats on chromosome 19.

FEATURES

- Inability of muscle relaxation.
- Early-onset cataract: Polychromatic opacities on the lens resembling a 'Christmas tree' cataract.
- Ptosis.
- Ophthalmoplegia.

7.9 KEARNS-SAYRE SYNDROME

Mitochondrial inherited myopathy due to deletion of mitochondrial DNA. Histopathology reveals 'ragged red fibres' due to increased intramuscular accumulation of mitochondria. It presents within the first two decades of life with a triad of:

- Bilateral, symmetrical ptosis and ophthalmoplegia.
- Pigmentary retinopathy with 'salt and pepper' appearance involving the macula.
- Cardiac conduction defects.

7.10 MILLER FISHER SYNDROME

A rare variant of Guillain-Barre syndrome. Anti-GQ1b antibodies may be present. It presents with a tetrad of ataxia, areflexia, ophthalmoplegia and facial diplegia.

7.11 NEUROFIBROMATOSIS TYPE 1

Neurofibromatosis type 1 (NF1) is an AD multisystem genetic disorder due to a mutation in the Neurofibromin 1 gene on chromosome 17.

FEATURES

- Café-au-lait spots: Brownish spots most commonly found on the trunk.
- Axillary freckling.
- Ophthalmic
  - Optic nerve glioma.
  - Bilateral Lisch nodules (iris hamartomas).

- Plexiform neurofibromas: 'Bag of worms' sensation in the eyelids
- Choroidal naevi: Patients with this have a higher risk of choroidal melanoma

7.12 NEUROFIBROMATOSIS TYPE 2

Neurofibromatosis type 2 (NF2) is less common than NF1. It occurs as a result of a mutation to the Neurofibromin 2 gene on chromosome 22.

FEATURES

- Posterior subcapsular cataracts.
- Bilateral/unilateral acoustic neuromas causing decreased sensorineural hearing loss, tinnitus and loss of corneal reflex.
- Meningiomas.

7.13 TUBEROUS SCLEROSIS

AD multisystem disorder characterized by the following.

- Facial angiofibroma.
- Ash-leaf spots: Hypopigmented macules on the skin.
- Seizures.
- Cognitive impairment.
- Multiple intracranial and/or retinal astrocytic hamartomas
  - Glial tumours of retinal fibre layer that arise from astrocytes.
  - They are commonly referred to as mulberry lesions due to their multinodular appearance. On fundoscopy they appear as well-defined elevated creamy white lesions.
  - Associations
    - Tuberous sclerosis (most common association)
    - Neurofibromatosis
    - Retinitis pigmentosa (less common; lesions are non-calcified)

7.14 BENIGN ESSENTIAL BLEPHAROSPASM

A bilateral idiopathic condition characterized by involuntary contraction of the orbicularis oculi muscle due to basal ganglia dysfunction. Presentation is in the sixth decade of life, with a female predominance. Blepharospasm and oromandibular dystonia can occur together in Meige syndrome.

MANAGEMENT

- Artificial tears for dry eyes.
- Botulinum toxin injection to orbicularis oculi. Side effects: Ptosis, dry eye, diplopia, lagophthalmos and corneal exposure.
- Surgical myectomy if the above does not work.

REFERENCES

1. Ramat S, Leigh RJ, Zee DS, Optican LM. What clinical disorders tell us about the neural control of saccadic eye movements. *Brain.* 2006;130(1):10–35.
2. Thier P, Ilg UJ. The neural basis of smooth-pursuit eye movements. *Curr Opin Neurobiol.* 2005;15(6):645–52.
3. Beck RW, Cleary PA, Anderson MM Jr et al. A randomized, controlled trial of corticosteroids in the treatment of acute optic neuritis. *N Engl J Med.* 1992;326(9):581–8.
4. Spector RH. The pupils. In:Walker HK, Hall WD, Hurst JE (editors).*Clinical Methods: The History, Physical, and Laboratory Examinations*, 3rd ed. Butterworth; 1990: chapter 8.
5. Lam BL, Thompson HS, Corbett JJ. The prevalence of simple anisocoria. *Am J Ophthalmol.* 1987;104(1):69–73.
6. Manchandia AM, Demer JL. Sensitivity of the three-step test in diagnosis of superior oblique palsy. *J Am Assoc Pediatr Ophthalmol Strabismus.* 2014;18(6):567–71.

8

Cornea

MOSTAFA KHALIL, OMAR KOULI AND RIZWAN MALIK

8.1 ANATOMY

The cornea and the sclera form the outermost fibrous layer of the eye. The cornea meets the sclera at the limbus. However, unlike the sclera, the cornea is a transparent structure.

8.1.1 Basics of the cornea

- Highest refraction power in the eye: 40 D.
- Refractive index: 1.376.
- Average diameter: 10–13 mm in adults and 9.5–10.5 mm in newborns.
- Thickness: It is about 535 μm thick centrally and thicker towards the periphery (660 μm).

8.1.2 Nutrient and nerve supply to the cornea

The cornea is an avascular structure; it receives most of its nutrients from the aqueous humour posteriorly and some from the tear film anteriorly. It is a highly sensitive structure, receiving sensory supply from CNV_1 via the long ciliary nerves.

8.1.3 Layers of the cornea

- Epithelial layer: Stratified nonkeratinized squamous epithelium. It has high regenerative potential to injury due to the presence of limbal epithelial stem cells (palisades of Vogt: prominent at superior and inferior limbus).
- Bowman layer: Avascular layer (no regeneration potential) that contains collagen fibres and terminates at the limbus.
- Stromal layer: The thickest corneal layer and is continuous with the sclera at the limbus. It is mainly made up of keratocytes and regularly orientated collagen fibrils (type I collagen). It can undergo scarring and has no regenerative potential.
- Descemet membrane: An elastic layer containing type IV collagen fibres.
- Endothelium: Functions by pumping excess fluid from the stroma to keep the cornea dehydrated to maintain its transparency.

8.2 BACTERIAL KERATITIS

Bacterial infection of the cornea is common and sight-threatening. It is more common in contact lens wearers (soft lenses > rigid lenses), especially with overnight wear and poor lens hygiene.

COMMON ORGANISMS

- *Pseudomonas aeruginosa* (most common cause of keratitis in contact lens wearers).
- *Staphylococcus aureus* and Streptococci infections.

FEATURES

- Unilateral sudden-onset pain, redness and photophobia with associated discharge and dVA.
- Purulent or mucopurulent discharge.
- Circumcorneal injection.
- White infiltrates epithelial and stromal involvement.
- Anterior chamber cells and hypopyon in severe keratitis.

COMPLICATIONS

Corneal perforation; this is more likely with the following organisms:

- *Neisseria gonorrhoeae*
- *Corynebacterium diphtheriae*
- *Haemophilus influenzae*

Table 8.1 Microorganisms and their correlating cultures and stains

Microorganisms	Media/stain
Most bacteria	Blood/chocolate agar and gram/Giemsa stain
Fungi	Sabouraud agar and gram/Giemsa stain
Mycobacterium	Ziehl-Neelsen stain and Lowenstein Jensen medium
Acanthamoeba	Non-nutrient agar with *Escherichia coli*

INVESTIGATIONS

Corneal scraping for microbiology. Table 8.1 summarizes cultures and stains used for different organisms.

MANAGEMENT

Topical broad-spectrum antibiotic treatment should be initiated even before laboratory results come back. Fluoroquinolones (e.g. ofloxacin) are typically used.

8.3 FUNGAL KERATITIS

Candida is a common cause of fungal keratitis in patients who are immunocompromised (AIDS, diabetics or on immunosuppressant such as steroids). Filamentous fungi such as *Aspergillus* or *Fusarium* are more common in patients who have had ocular trauma, classically from contaminated plant matter or a tree branch.

Fungal infections usually present with unilateral redness, tearing and blurred vision. Usually, patients will complain of mild pain and photophobia. Specific signs for different organisms are:

- *Candida*: Small ulcer with an expanding infiltrate in a 'collar stud' formation.
- Filamentous: Feathery branching-like infiltrate pattern.

Investigations are the same as bacterial keratitis (Table 8.1); however, confocal microscopy can aid with quick diagnosis.

MANAGEMENT
- Natamycin drops for proven filamentous.
- Voriconazole or amphotericin B drops for proven *Candida*.

8.4 *ACANTHAMOEBA* KERATITIS

A type of keratitis caused by the organism *Acanthamoeba*. Risk factors stem from improper lens hygiene (showering/swimming in contact lenses).

FEATURES
- Patients usually present with pain that is out of proportion to clinical signs, with associated photophobia and blurred vision.

- In early disease, the signs are usually mild and not specific to *Acanthamoeba*. However, in late disease, perineural infiltrates and ring-shaped stromal infiltrates can be seen.

INVESTIGATION AND MANAGEMENT

Corneal scraping (Table 8.1) and/or confocal microscopy to identify the presence of amoebic cysts. Keratitis is usually treated with topical polyhexamethylene biguanide or chlorhexidine.

8.5 HERPES SIMPLEX KERATITIS

Herpes simplex virus (HSV) is a double-stranded DNA virus. Primary infection results in blepharoconjunctivitis. The virus usually remains latent in the trigeminal ganglion. Reactivation usually results in recurrent keratitis. Keratitis may affect the epithelial, stromal or endothelial layers of the cornea.

8.5.1 Epithelial keratitis

Reactivation of the HSV presents with pain, dVA, lacrimation and foreign body sensation.

SIGNS

- Superficial punctate keratitis which causes a stellate (star-shaped) erosion which later becomes a *classic dendritic ulcer* (Figure 8.1) which can be clearly seen with fluorescein. (*Note*: Epithelial cells at the dendrite margin stain well with rose Bengal.)
- Reduced corneal sensation.

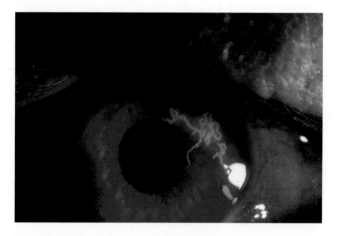

Figure 8.1 The dendritic ulcer in HSV keratitis.

8.5.2 Disciform keratitis (endothelial)

This form usually occurs from HSV antigen hypersensitivity, rather than reactivation. Presentation is with insidious onset of painless dVA.

SIGNS

- Central circular stromal oedema
- There is usually mild anterior chamber activity
- Keratitic precipitates
- Wessely ring (Figure 8.2): Antigen/antibody complex

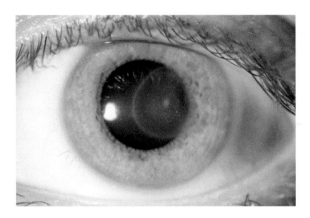

Figure 8.2 Wessely ring in HSV disciform keratitis.

INVESTIGATIONS

Diagnosis is mainly clinical; however, it can be aided by corneal swabs for PCR or Giemsa staining which shows multinuclear giant cells.

MANAGEMENT

- Epithelial
  - Topical acyclovir.
  - Avoid steroids: May lead to geographic ulcer and corneal perforation.
- Disciform
  - Oral acyclovir 400 mg five times a day.
  - Avoid topical steroids until epithelium is intact. Use the lowest effective dose of dexamethasone or prednisolone if indicated.

8.6 HERPES ZOSTER OPHTHALMICUS

Herpes zoster ophthalmicus (HZO) infection is caused by varicella zoster virus (VZV). Primary infection usually leads to chickenpox. However, reactivation leads to shingles (herpes zoster) of the affected dermatome. Thus, HZO refers to shingles affecting the dermatome supplied by CNV_1.

CUTANEOUS FEATURES

- Rash (vesicles or papules).
- Painful neuralgia.
- Hutchinson sign: Involvement of the tip of the nose. Indicates a higher likelihood for ocular disease due to the involvement of the nasociliary nerve.

OPHTHALMIC FEATURES

- Epithelial keratitis: Pseudo-dendrites are the differentiating feature from HSV keratitis. These are usually grey, not ulcerated, with less branching and lacking in terminal bulbs. These stain poorly with fluorescein.
- Conjunctivitis.
- Elevated IOP.
- Stromal and disciform keratitis are less common.

MANAGEMENT

- Oral acyclovir 800 mg five times a day.
- Amitriptyline for neuropathic pain.

8.7 INTERSTITIAL KERATITIS (IK)

This is not a diagnosis but rather a sign of underlying pathology. It describes stromal inflammation ± neovascularization. It is caused by the invasion of microorganism or an immune reaction to a foreign antigen.

FEATURES

- Pain, dVA and photophobia.
- Non-ulcerated stromal keratitis characterized by feathery mid-stromal scarring with ghost vessels.

AETIOLOGY

- Syphilis
  - Congenital disease usually causes bilateral corneal involvement, while acquired disease is usually unilateral.
  - Hutchinson triad of congenital syphilis (late feature): Interstitial keratitis, notched teeth and sensorineural deafness.
  - Treatment: IM benzylpenicillin and topical steroids.
- Lyme disease
  - Caused by the spirochete bacteria *Borrelia*, which is transmitted to humans via a tick bite.
  - Causes erythema migrans (bull's-eye skin rash), arthralgia, facial palsy, loss of temporal eyebrows and interstitial keratitis.
- Viral: HSV and VZV, Epstein–Barr virus (EBV).

- Cogan syndrome
  - Autoimmune disorder.
  - Interstitial keratitis with sensorineural hearing loss, vertigo and tinnitus.
  - Complications: Polyarteritis nodosa.

8.8 MARGINAL KERATITIS

A type of peripheral corneal inflammation due to a type III hypersensitivity reaction to staphylococcal exotoxin, mainly *Staphylococcus aureus*. Associated with rosacea and blepharitis.

FEATURES

- Epiphora, redness and photophobia.
- Chronic blepharitis.
- Subepithelial infiltrates separated from the limbus by a clear zone.
- Typically occurs in regions where the eyelid contacts the cornea.

MANAGEMENT

Lid hygiene and mild topical steroids.

8.9 PERIPHERAL ULCERATIVE KERATITIS

Peripheral ulcerative keratitis (PUK) is a group of conditions that leads to peripheral corneal thinning. The most common systemic association is rheumatoid arthritis. Other associations include polyarteritis nodosa, Wegener granulomatosis and relapsing polychondritis.

FEATURES

- The disease usually begins peripherally, but eventually progresses centrally and posteriorly. End stage is a thin vascular cornea.
- Interpalpebral peripheral corneal stromal thinning with an epithelial defect.
- Episcleritis and/or scleritis may be present.

MANAGEMENT

Oral prednisolone ± systemic immunosuppression. Note that topical steroids may exacerbate the thinning.

8.10 OCULAR ROSACEA

Acne rosacea leads to facial skin changes and ocular disease (Figure 8.3). It causes telangiectasia, papules and pustules on the face, facial flushing and rhinophyma.

OCULAR FEATURES

- Dry eyes, redness, epiphora and photophobia
- Eyelids: Telangiectasia and posterior blepharitis
- Conjunctival hyperaemia

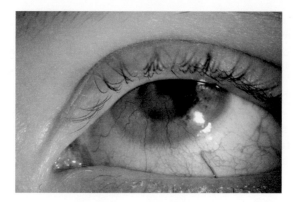

Figure 8.3 Ocular rosacea with eyelid telangiectasia and peripheral corneal vascularization.

- Cornea
  - Marginal keratitis
  - Inferior corneal thinning
  - Superficial erosions
  - Peripheral corneal vascularization

MANAGEMENT
- Lid hygiene and hot compression
- Topical lubricants
- Oral tetracycline

8.11 FILAMENTARY KERATITIS

This is a condition in which the corneal epithelium degenerates, leading strands/filaments and mucus to adhere to the corneal surface.

RISK FACTORS

Anything that leads to changes in the tear film or corneal surface:

- Dry eye syndrome
- Corneal epithelium erosions
- Laser eye surgery
- Contact lens wear

FEATURES
- The main presenting feature is foreign body sensation.
- Redness, epiphora and blepharospasm and dry eyes.
- 'Comma-shaped' lesions (strands of epithelial cells) that move up and down on blinking which stains well with rose bengal stains.

8.12 KERATOCONUS

This is a bilateral and asymmetrical condition characterized by progressive central stromal thinning and apical protrusion of the cornea, usually presenting in early adulthood.

ASSOCIATIONS

- Down syndrome
- Marfan syndrome
- Ehlers-Danlos syndrome
- Leber congenital amaurosis
- Retinitis pigmentosa
- History of atopy

FEATURES

- Irregular astigmatism.
- Lower eyelid protrusion on downgaze (Munson sign).
- Vertical striations in the stroma, seen on slit lamp (Vogt striae).
- Iron deposit often within the epithelium around the base of the cone (Fleischer ring).
- 'Oil drop' reflex on ophthalmoscopy.
- 'Scissoring' reflex on retinoscopy.

COMPLICATION

Acute hydrops

- Tear in Descemet membrane leading to corneal oedema.
- Presentation: dVA, pain and photophobia.

INVESTIGATIONS

- Keratometry: Grading of keratoconus, into mild, moderate and severe; <48D = mild and >54D = severe.
- Video keratography (corneal topography): Essential to pick up early keratoconus. Very useful for monitoring and has replaced keratometry. It shows an asymmetrical 'bow-tie' pattern in early disease and progresses into a steep cone that is displaced off the visual axis.

MANAGEMENT

- Mild: Spectacle correction.
- Moderate: Rigid/hard contact lenses or corneal collagen cross-linking using riboflavin drops and ultraviolet-A.
- Severe: Penetrating or deep anterior lamellar keratoplasty.
- LASIK is generally contraindicated.

8.13 MICROPHTHALMIA

A condition in which the whole eye is smaller than the average by at least two standard deviations.

- Simple microphthalmos (nanophthalmos)
  - Bilateral involvement; the eye is small but otherwise normal.
  - Associated with angle-closure glaucoma, uveal effusion syndrome, hypermetropia, amblyopia and strabismus.
- Complex microphthalmos
  - A small eye associated with other abnormalities including orbital cysts or colobomas (hole in ocular structure).
  - Associated with fetal alcohol syndrome and intrauterine infections.

8.14 WILSON DISEASE

An AR genetic disorder causing deposition of copper in the body. The most common areas affected are the liver, brain and eyes.

FEATURES

- Hepatic cirrhosis leading to portal hypertension, ascites, varices and hepatic encephalopathy.
- Movement disorders and ataxia.
- Kayser-Fleischer ring: Copper deposition in Descemet's membrane.
- Anterior subcapsular sunflower cataracts.

8.15 BAND KERATOPATHY

This is not a diagnosis but a sign due to calcium deposition in the Bowman's layer.

AETIOLOGY

- Idiopathic
- Old age
- Hypercalcemia and hyperphosphatemia (renal failure)
- Silicone oil
- Chronic anterior uveitis

FEATURES

- Often asymptomatic.
- Interpalpebral peripheral zone calcification (band-like chalky plaque) with a clear zone separating it from the limbus.

MANAGEMENT

- Treat underlying cause.
- Chelation with ethylenediaminetetraacetic acid (EDTA).

8.16 CORNEAL DYSTROPHIES

A group of progressive, hereditary disorders that cause corneal opacification and can lead to visual impairment. They can be classified as anterior (predominantly affecting the epithelium), stromal or endothelial.

8.16.1 Anterior dystrophies

In this book, we discuss a select few: Cogan and Reis-Buckler dystrophies.

8.16.1.1 COGAN DYSTROPHY (MAP-DOT-FINGERPRINT DYSTROPHY)

This is the most common epithelial dystrophy. Sporadic or AD inheritance.

Features

Onset is normally in the second decade with bilateral recurrent corneal erosions (recurrent pain, photophobia and epiphora). Signs are best seen on retroillumination slit lamp.

- Map: Subepithelial geographic opacities
- Dot: Intraepithelial microcysts
- Fingerprint: Subepithelial ridges

8.16.1.2 REIS-BUCKLER DYSTROPHY

An AD condition that occurs as a result of the replacement of Bowman's layer with connective tissue.

Features

Presents with recurrent corneal erosions in childhood. These become less painful with age due to decreased corneal sensation. Examination may reveal subepithelial cloudy opacities centrally.

8.16.2 Stromal dystrophies

Three important types: lattice dystrophy, granular dystrophy and macular dystrophy are discussed. The mnemonic 'Marilyn Monroe Always Gets Her Men in LA County' is useful to help remember the features of these conditions.

8.16.2.1 MACULAR DYSTROPHY

'Marilyn Monroe Always': *M*acular dystrophy, *M*ucopolysaccharide accumulation in the stroma, *A*lcian blue is used to stain the mucopolysaccharides.

Features

- Bilateral visual loss in the first decade of life.
- Grey, poorly demarcated opacities in the stroma.

8.16.2.2 GRANULAR DYSTROPHY

'Gets Her Men': Granular dystrophy, Hyaline deposits in the stroma, Masson trichome is used to stain hyaline.

Features

- dVA and recurrent corneal erosions.
- Breadcrumb-like opacities in an otherwise healthy stroma.

8.16.2.3 LATTICE DYSTROPHY

'LA County': Lattice dystrophy, Amyloid deposits in the stroma, Congo red is used to stain amyloid (showing green birefringence on polarized light).

Features

- dVA and recurrent corneal erosions.
- Reduced corneal sensation.
- Examination shows anterior glassy stromal dots, affecting the centre, form together to form fine filamentous lines.

8.16.3 Endothelial dystrophies

8.16.3.1 FUCHS' ENDOTHELIAL DYSTROPHY

The most common corneal dystrophy. Inheritance is sporadic or AD. It is more common in elderly females. It is due to a failure of the Na^+K^+ pump leading to accumulation of fluid in the cornea which leads to endothelial cell loss.

Features

- Blurry vision worse in the morning.
- Specular microscopy may show corneal guttata ('beaten metal' appearance) and low endothelial cell counts.
- Pachymetry may show increased central corneal thickness (CCT).

9

Conjunctiva

OMAR KOULI, MOSTAFA KHALIL AND RIZWAN MALIK

9.1 ANATOMY

The conjunctiva is a translucent mucous membrane that covers the anterior globe and terminates at the corneoscleral limbus. The conjunctiva is continuous with the skin at the eyelid margin. It is made of three parts:

1. Palpebral conjunctiva: Starts at the mucocutaneous transitional zone of the lid margin and is strongly adherent to the posterior aspect of the tarsal plates.
2. Forniceal conjunctiva: A loose fold made by the conjunctiva, covering the posterior eyelid and anterior surface of the eyeball.
3. Bulbar conjunctiva: The thinnest part, covering the anterior surface of the sclera. It is loosely attached, except at the limbus where it is fused with underlying sclera and Tenon's capsule.

9.1.1 Nerve supply

The conjunctiva is mainly supplied by CNV1. However, the infraorbital nerve supplies a part of the inferior conjunctiva. The limbus is supplied by the long ciliary nerve, a branch of the nasociliary nerve.

9.1.2 Blood supply

The peripheral and marginal arterial arcades of the eyelids supply the palpebral and forniceal part of the conjunctiva. The bulbar part is supplied by the posterior (from arterial arcades of the eyelid) and anterior (from the anterior ciliary artery) conjunctival arteries.

9.1.3 Lymphatic drainage

The medial part of the conjunctiva drains to the submandibular lymph nodes, while the lateral part drains to the preauricular lymph nodes.

9.2 ACUTE BACTERIAL CONJUNCTIVITIS

Bacterial conjunctivitis may take an acute or chronic course. Pathogens for acute bacterial conjunctivitis include *Streptococcus pneumoniae*, *Staphylococcus aureus*, *Haemophilus influenzae* and, rarely, *Neisseria gonorrhoeae*.

FEATURES

- Unilateral initially but becomes sequentially bilateral.
- Redness, grittiness and purulent discharge.
- Patients may complain of a 'sticky eye' upon awakening.
- Hyperaemia (conjunctival injection).
- Gonococcal disease is typically more severe and hyperacute. Associated with lid oedema, severe mucopurulent discharge and lymphadenopathy. (*Note*: Lymphadenopathy is not present in typical bacterial conjunctivitis.)

TREATMENT

Most cases are self-limiting. If severe, treat with topical chloramphenicol or fusidic acid.

9.3 ADULT INCLUSION (CHLAMYDIAL) CONJUNCTIVITIS

This infection is caused by the serological variants D–K of *Chlamydia trachomatis*. It causes a subacute onset of unilateral conjunctivitis; if left untreated, it may follow a chronic course.

FEATURES

- Red eye with mucopurulent discharge.
- Preauricular lymphadenopathy.

- Follicles (whitish, round and discrete swellings) are present, most commonly in the inferior fornix.
- Epithelial keratitis and subepithelial corneal infiltrates may occur.
- Reiter syndrome: Urethritis + arthritis + conjunctivitis/anterior uveitis.

INVESTIGATIONS

- Giemsa stain: Basophilic intracytoplasmic inclusion bodies.
- Direct immunofluorescent staining: Free elementary bodies.
- Swab for culturing (McCoy).

TREATMENT

1 g oral azithromycin single dose or 100 mg doxycycline twice a day for 14 days.

9.4 TRACHOMA

Trachoma is the leading cause of infectious blindness worldwide. Trachoma is caused by serological variants A–C of C. trachomatis.

- Transmission: Musca sorbens fly acts as a vector.
- Risk factors: Poverty and poor hygiene.

PATHOPHYSIOLOGY

A type IV hypersensitivity reaction. Trachomatous disease is split into two parts: an active inflammatory phase and a cicatricial (scarring) chronic phase. The recurrence of active inflammation to the eye leads to scarring, trichiasis and eventual blindness as a result of corneal damage due to eyelashes irritating the cornea.

EPIDEMIOLOGY (1)

- The most trachoma-endemic continent is Africa.
- The highest prevalence is in Ethiopia.
- Number of global visually impaired or blind: 1.9 million people.
- Women are four times more likely to require surgery for trichiasis.

WHO STAGING (2)

1. Trachomatous inflammation-follicular (TF): 5+ follicles present in the upper tarsal conjunctiva.
2. Trachomatous inflammation-intense (TI): Upper tarsal conjunctiva is thickened, and the majority of the blood vessels are obscured.
3. Trachomatous scarring (TS): Conjunctival scarring (cicatricial).
4. Trachomatous trichiasis (TT): Ingrowth of eyelashes towards the cornea.
5. Corneal opacity (CO): Due to eyelashes rubbing on the cornea.

ACTIVE INFLAMMATORY PHASE

- Follicular conjunctivitis: Most prominent in the superior tarsal plate. May be associated with papillae (red, elevated dots with a vascularized centre).
- Vascularization of the superior cornea (pannus formation).

CHRONIC CICATRICIAL PHASE

- Herbert pits: Shallow depressions in the superior limbus created by follicles (pathognomonic for trachoma).
- Arlt's line: Conjunctival scars.
- Trichiasis, entropion and eventual corneal opacities may eventually develop.

MANAGEMENT

WHO 'SAFE' strategy (2):

- **S**urgery for trichiasis: Bilamellar tarsal rotation surgery can be performed to correct trichiasis.
- **A**ntibiotics: Single dose of 1 g oral azithromycin.
- **F**acial cleanliness.
- **E**nvironmental improvement.

9.5 OPHTHALMIA NEONATORUM

Ophthalmia neonatorum is defined as conjunctival inflammation developing in the first 30 days of life. Table 9.1 summarizes the common causative microorganisms.

9.6 VIRAL CONJUNCTIVITIS

The most common causative agent is adenovirus (Table 9.2). Other viruses include herpes simplex and *Molluscum contagiosum*.

Table 9.1 Causes of ophthalmia neonatorum

Microorganism	Features	Onset	Management
Chlamydia (most common cause)	Mucopurulent discharge and papillary conjunctivitis	1–3 weeks	Oral erythromycin
Gonococcal	Hyperpurulent discharge, eyelid swelling ± corneal ulcer	1–3 days	IM ceftriaxone
HSV	Watery discharge, periocular skin vesicles and dendritic corneal epithelial lesion	1–2 weeks	IV acyclovir
Staphylococci	Purulent discharge and mild sticky eye	1 week	Topical chloramphenicol

Table 9.2 Types of viral conjunctivitis

Subtypes	Acute nonspecific follicular conjunctivitis (ANFC)	Pharyngoconjunctival fever (PCF)	Epidemic keratoconjunctivitis (EKC)
Background	This is the most commonly seen type	Due to adenoviral serotypes 3, 4 and 7	Due to adenoviral serotypes 8, 19 and 37

Features	• Red, itchy, gritty eye with associated watery discharge
	• Starts unilateral but progresses to bilateral involvement after a couple of days
	• Follicular conjunctivitis with conjunctival hyperaemia
	• Preauricular lymphadenopathy
		• Fever
		• Pharyngitis
		• Conjunctivitis (similar to ANFC)
		• Lymphadenopathy
		• Keratitis
			• Conjunctivitis (similar to ANFC)
			• Keratitis:
			  • Occurs after conjunctivitis
			  • Characterized by epithelial microcysts (early) and punctate epithelial keratitis (late)
			  • More common in EKC than in PCF

9.7 ALLERGIC CONJUNCTIVITIS

The four subtypes of allergic conjunctivitis discussed are:

1. Seasonal and perennial allergic conjunctivitis
2. Vernal keratoconjunctivitis (VKC)
3. Atopic keratoconjunctivitis (AKC)
4. Giant papillary conjunctivitis

9.7.1 Seasonal and perennial allergic conjunctivitis

1. Seasonal: IgE-mediated type I hypersensitivity. Worse during spring and summer.
2. Perennial: IgE-mediated type I hypersensitivity. All year round when exposed to allergens.

FEATURES
- Red, watery and itchy eye.
- May be associated with rhinitis.
- Conjunctival hyperaemia and papillary conjunctivitis.

TREATMENT
- Avoid allergens
- Artificial tears
- Topical/oral antihistamines
- Topical sodium cromoglicate

9.7.2 Vernal keratoconjunctivitis (VKC) and atopic keratoconjunctivitis (AKC)

Both VKC and AKC affect conjunctiva, eyelids and the cornea (Table 9.3). They are both bilateral conditions, expressing IgE-mediated (type I hypersensitivity) and T-cell-mediated (type IV hypersensitivity) immune responses. Symptoms are characterized by itching, discharge, blepharospasm and photophobia.

MANAGEMENT
- Avoid allergens
- Artificial tears
- Topical/oral antihistamines
- Topical cromoglicate
- Topical ciclosporin
- Topical steroids

9.7.3 Giant papillary conjunctivitis

A type I and IV hypersensitivity reaction to contact lens wear. Patients usually complain of increased ocular tiredness while wearing contact lenses. This is

Table 9.3 VKC versus AKC

Condition	VKC	AKC
Background	• Onset: <10 years old • Boys > girls • 5% may develop AKC • Common in dry, warm climates and is usually seasonal • Eosinophils present	• Onset: In adults • No gender predominance • Association: History of atopic dermatitis • Follows a more chronic course than VKC
Conjunctiva	• Superior tarsus involved • Conjunctival hyperaemia • 'Stringy' mucous discharge • Macropapillae (flat-topped polygonal dots with 'cobblestone' appearance), can progress to giant papillae (>1 mm)	• Inferior tarsus involved • Conjunctival hyperaemia • Watery discharge • Papillae are typically smaller than VKC initially
Limbus	• Horner-Trantas dots: White dots of accumulated eosinophils • Gelatinous papillae	• Similar to VKC
Cornea	• Superior punctate epithelial erosions • 'Shield' ulcers: Mucous and calcium phosphate accumulation in Bowman's membrane • Keratoconus may occur due to repeated eye rubbing	• Punctate epithelial erosion inferiorly • Vascularization and scarring more common than VKC • Keratoconus may occur due to repeated eye rubbing.
Eyelids	Mild involvement	• More significant than in VKC • Shows eczematous skin changes • Chronic anterior staphylococcal blepharitis

associated with pruritus, red eye and mucous secretion, which may be worse after taking off the lenses.

SIGNS

- Superior tarsal hyperaemia.
- Superior tarsal papillae (classically 'giant' >1 mm; however, size is not necessary for diagnosis).

MANAGEMENT

Discontinue contact lens wear.

9.8 OCULAR MUCOUS MEMBRANE PEMPHIGOID

This is a chronic, blistering autoimmune disease. It has a type II hypersensitivity response to autoantibodies attacking the basement membrane. Typically, elderly females are affected.

FEATURES

- Bilateral conjunctivitis with conjunctival hyperaemia, swelling and subepithelial fibrosis (mostly seen in inferior fornix), associated with reduced inferior forniceal depth.
- Symblepharon: Union of the palpebral and bulbar conjunctiva.
- Dry eyes due to goblet cell destruction.
- Trichiasis.
- Chronic blepharitis.
- Ankyloblepharon: Union of lateral canthus and both eyelids.
- Keratinization, vascularization and epithelial defects of the cornea may ensue.

INVESTIGATION

Direct conjunctival immunofluorescence: linear bands of IgG and IgA deposits at the basement membrane.

TREATMENT

Dapsone can be used for mild disease. Other immunomodulatory agents (e.g. azathioprine and methotrexate) can be used for more severe cases. Corticosteroids are useful for severe acute cases.

9.9 SUPERIOR LIMBIC KERATOCONJUNCTIVITIS

Superior limbic keratoconjunctivitis (SLK) is an idiopathic chronic inflammatory condition affecting the superior bulbar conjunctiva, limbus and cornea. It is more common in females and there appears to be a strong association with TED. There is also an association with sicca syndrome and rheumatoid arthritis.

FEATURES

Gradual-onset foreign body, burning and itching with associated photophobia and pain. On examination, there is:

- Localized conjunctival hyperaemia and papillary reaction superiorly.
- Occasionally, thickening of the superior bulbar conjunctiva is seen. This stains with fluorescein and rose bengal stains.
- Cornea may be affected with superior punctate epithelial erosions and filamentary keratitis.

9.10 PARINAUD OCULOGLANDULAR SYNDROME

This is a rare condition caused by various bacterial, fungal and viral agents, most notably *Bartonella henselae* (cat scratch disease). The syndrome is characterized by a granulomatous unilateral conjunctivitis with ipsilateral preauricular lymphadenopathy associated with a low-grade fever.

9.11 PINGUECULA

Bulbar conjunctival degeneration characterized by a yellow/white patch most commonly on the nasal limbus. It never grows over the cornea. Risk factors include ultraviolet light exposure and ageing.

9.12 PTERYGIUM

Bulbar conjunctival degeneration characterized by a pink fleshy triangular-shaped fibrovascular wedge (Figure 9.1). Usually arises on the nasal limbus, causing destruction of Bowman's layer, and grows over the cornea.

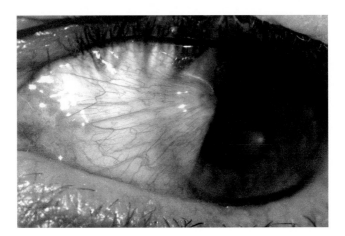

Figure 9.1 A pterygium encroaching on the cornea.

Possible complications include obscuring the optical access and causing astigmatism. Risk factors are ultraviolet light and dry climates.

FEATURES

- Stocker's line: Epithelial iron deposits in the cornea.
- Fuchs' islets: Small white dots in the cornea.
- May cause ocular dryness, astigmatism or reduced vision (if within visual axis).

MANAGEMENT

Conservative management (reassurance, lubrication) or surgical excision for cosmesis or for visual interference. However, it should be noted that recurrence is high.

REFERENCES

1. International Coalition for Trachoma Control. Key Trachoma Facts and Statistics. http://www.trachomacoalition.org/about-trachoma.
2. World Health Organization. Trachoma. https://www.who.int/trachoma/en/.

10

Sclera

OMAR KOULI, MOSTAFA KHALIL AND RIZWAN MALIK

10.1 ANATOMY

The sclera forms 5/6 of the outer coat of the globe. It starts at the limbus anteriorly and terminates at the optic nerve posteriorly. The sclera is thinnest posterior to the rectus muscle insertion and thickest surrounding the optic nerve.

There are three parts to the sclera:

1. Episclera (outermost): Thin vascularized connective tissue anterior to the sclera and posterior to the Tenon capsule.
2. Substantia propria: Made of irregularly arranged type I collagen fibrils.
3. Lamina fusca (innermost): Made of loosely arranged connective tissue and separated from the choroid by the suprachoroidal space.

INNERVATION

- Anterior sclera: Long posterior ciliary nerves.
- Posterior sclera: Short posterior ciliary nerves.

10.2 EPISCLERITIS

Episcleritis (inflammation of the episclera) is a common self-limiting condition which typically affects middle-aged females. It is usually idiopathic.

SIMPLE EPISCLERITIS

- Most common.
- Acute onset, peaking at 12–24 hours and then slowly fades after a few days.
- Localized triangular redness and discomfort.

NODULAR EPISCLERITIS

- Insidious onset and longer recovery time.
- Red eye and discomfort are the most common symptoms.
- Tender vascular nodule seen most commonly at the interpalpebral fissure.

INVESTIGATION

Instillation of 10% phenylephrine blanches the redness in episcleritis.

MANAGEMENT

Cool compresses and oral nonsteroidal anti-inflammatory drugs (NSAIDs).

10.3 SCLERITIS

Full-thickness inflammation of the sclera, most commonly associated with autoimmune diseases.

SYSTEMIC ASSOCIATIONS

- Rheumatoid arthritis (RA): The most common systemic association of scleritis. (*Note*: The most common ocular manifestation of RA is keratoconjunctivitis sicca.)
- Granulomatosis with polyangiitis.
- Polyarteritis nodosa.
- Relapsing polychondritis.
- Infection: Herpes zoster, Lyme disease, syphilis, etc.

10.3.1 Anterior scleritis

DIFFUSE

- Most common.
- Dull pain that may radiate to the forehead or jaw.
- Gradual onset of localized or diffuse redness of the eye.
- Oedematous sclera that often resolves leaving a bluish hue (due to scleral translucency).

NODULAR

- Gradual onset of pain followed by red eye.
- Single or multiple erythematous, tender nodules.

NECROTIZING SCLERITIS WITH INFLAMMATION

- Most severe form, can result in visual loss.
- Subacute severe ocular pain that radiates to the forehead or jaw.
- Redness and lacrimation.
- White patches of scleral oedema that block overlying episclera and conjunctiva vasculature, leading to low perfusion and necrosis to scleral tissue.

SCLEROMALACIA PERFORANS

- Also known as necrotizing scleritis without inflammation.
- Bilateral involvement, typically seen in elderly patients with advanced RA.
- Characterized by an asymptomatic, gradual onset of necrotic patches leading to scleral thinning exposing the underlying uvea.

MANAGEMENT

- Instillation of 10% phenylephrine does not blanch vessels in scleritis.
- Oral NSAIDs for mild-moderate scleritis.
- Systemic steroids and/or other immunomodulatory therapy for severe or necrotizing scleritis.

10.3.2 Posterior scleritis

Posterior scleritis is a rare inflammatory condition affecting the posterior sclera.

FEATURES

- Severe pain (not correlating with severity of inflammation)
- Choroidal folds
- Retinal detachment
- Diplopia and mild proptosis
- Optic disc swelling and vision loss

INVESTIGATIONS

B-scan ultrasound shows increased thickness of the sclera and fluid accumulation in the sub-Tenon space giving rise to a characteristic 'T' sign.

MANAGEMENT

Oral NSAIDs ± corticosteroids.

10.4 BLUE SCLERA

A blue sclera is a result of exposure of underlying uvea due to scleral thinning.

SYSTEMIC ASSOCIATIONS

- Osteogenesis imperfecta
  - AD inherited disease as a result of type I collagen defects. Characterized by fragility fractures, short stature, hearing loss and easy bruising.
  - Ocular features: Blue sclera, megalocornea and shallow orbits.
- Ehlers-Danlos syndrome
  - AR inherited condition characterized by joint laxity, cardiovascular problems and easy bruising.
  - Ocular features: Blue sclera, keratoconus, lens subluxation and strabismus.

11

Lens and cataracts

AHMED HASSANE AND STEWART GILLAN

11.1 ANATOMY AND PHYSIOLOGY

The lens is a biconvex crystalline structure located between the iris and vitreous. It has a power of 15–20D in adults and 43–47D in infancy. Its high-protein (crystalline) content gives the lens a high refractive index of about 1.4.

11.1.1 Accommodation

- Near: The eye brings near objects into focus by contracting the ciliary muscle. This results in the relaxation of the zonules making the lens more spherical and increasing its diopter power.
- Far: The eye brings far objects into focus by relaxing the ciliary muscle. This increases zonular tension, making the lens flat.

11.1.2 Histology

CAPSULE
- An outer transparent basement membrane.
- Thinnest posteriorly and thickest near the equators.
- Made of type IV collagen and glycosaminoglycan.
- Anterior capsule thickens with age, but the posterior capsule maintains the same thickness.

EPITHELIUM
- Simple cuboidal cells located beneath the capsule.
- Central zone: Present on the anterior surface of the lens.
- Pre-equatorial zone: Cells undergo mitotic division throughout life and form the lens fibres.
- No epithelium on the posterior surface of the lens.

LENS FIBRES
- Lens fibres elongate, pushing the older fibres deeper into the lens.
- The nucleus is the innermost part, which is present at birth, and the cortex is the outer part, which contains the youngest fibres.
- The junction of lens fibres forms sutures:
  - Anterior suture: Has an upright Y-shaped suture.
  - Posterior suture: Has an inverted Y-shaped suture.

ZONULES
Suspensory ligaments, made of fibrillin, attached to the lens equator.

11.2 CATARACT MATURITY

A cataract is the progressive cloudiness of the lens causing gradual vision loss and blindness if untreated. It is the leading cause of blindness worldwide.

GRADE
- Immature cataract: Partially opaque.
- Mature cataract: Completely opaque.
- Hypermature cataract: Shrunken anterior capsule due to leakage of material outside the lens.
- Morgagnian cataract: A form of hypermature cataract with cortex liquefaction causing the nucleus to sink. Complications include phacoanaphylactic uveitis and phacolytic glaucoma.

11.3 AGE-RELATED CATARACTS

These are the most common type of cataracts and can be classified as nuclear, cortical, subcapsular and polychromatic cataracts.

11.3.1 Nuclear sclerotic

Characterized by the yellowing of the crystalline lens due to the deposition of the urochrome pigment.

It can cause a myopic shift leading to 'second sight' phenomenon. Due to the lens becoming harder, the refractive index increases, allowing for some elderly patients to read without glasses.

11.3.2 Cortical

Cortical cataracts occur due to the opacification of the lens cortex. Characterized by wedge-shaped opacities. Glare is the predominant symptom, especially from headlights while driving at night.

11.3.3 Subcapsular

- Anterior subcapsula: Opacities under the anterior capsule.
- Posterior subcapsular: Opacities under the posterior capsule. Glare is a common symptom. Patients may complain of difficulty seeing in bright light and near vision.

11.3.4 Polychromatic ('Christmas tree')

Characterized by needle-like opacities in the deep cortex and nucleus (Figure 11.1).

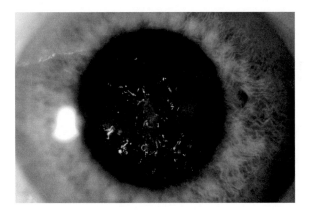

Figure 11.1 Polychromatic 'Christmas tree' cataract.

11.4 ACQUIRED CATARACTS AND THEIR ASSOCIATIONS

11.4.1 Anterior subcapsular

- Blunt trauma (flower-shaped cataract)
- Atopic dermatitis (shield-like cataract)

- Wilson disease (sunflower cataract)
- Post-congestive angle closure glaucoma (glaukomflecken)
- Gold (drug induced)
- Infrared radiation (glass-blower cataract)

11.4.2 Posterior subcapsular

- Corticosteroids
- Diabetes (snowflake shaped)
- Retinitis pigmentos
- NF2
- Chloroquine

11.4.3 Other cataracts

- Christmas tree-like cataract appearance: Myotonic dystrophy
- Pearly nuclear sclerotic cataract: Rubella
- Blue dot cataract: Down syndrome
- Polychromatic cataract: Hypoparathyroidism

11.5 MANAGEMENT

Cataract surgery involves the replacement of the diseased lens with an intraocular lens (IOL). This is achieved by:

- Phacoemulsification (gold standard): This technique uses an ultrasonically driven needle (phaco tip) to chop the nucleus and then aspirate the lens material.
- Extracapsular cataract extraction (ECCE): May be used for very hard cataracts.

11.5.1 Advantages of phacoemulsification over ECCE

- Smaller incision
- Less astigmatism
- Faster recovery
- Reduced complications
- No sutures needed

11.5.2 Intraocular lens power

IOL power is determined by measuring the curvature of the cornea and eye length. Power (P) is calculated using the following equation:

$$P = A - 2.5L - 0.9K \tag{11.1}$$

where:

- *A* is a constant supplied by the manufacturer.
- *L* is the axial length of the eye, measured using A-scan ultrasonography.
- *K* is the average corneal power reading in diopters.

11.5.3 Types of IOLs

RIGID IOL

- Made of polymethylmethacrylate (PMMA).
- Requires a larger incision.
- Higher rates of posterior capsular opacification (PCO) than flexible IOL.

FLEXIBLE IOL

- Used in modern cataract surgery.
- Three types
  - Acrylic hydrophobic IOL: Has a higher refractive index and lower rates of PCO than its hydrophilic counterparts. However, can cause dysphotopsia (troublesome glare).
  - Acrylic hydrophilic IOL: Has higher biocompatibility. However, calcification of the lens (causing lens opacities) may occur.
  - Silicone IOL: Less commonly used in modern phacoemulsification.

11.6 COMPLICATIONS OF SURGERY

- Intraoperative
  - Posterior lens capsule rupture.
  - Floppy iris syndrome: A flaccid iris that can complicate surgery. It usually occurs with some patients on alpha blockers (e.g. tamsulosin). Intracameral phenylephrine can be used to dilate pupils in high risk patients [1].
- Postoperative
  - Early: Corneal oedema, elevated IOP and acute endophthalmitis.
  - Late: PCO (most common complication), Irvine-Gass syndrome (CMO post cataract surgery), retinal detachment (especially in patients with high myopia) and delayed endophthalmitis.

11.6.1 Endophthalmitis

Endophthalmitis is the inflammation of the vitreous and aqueous humour, usually caused by infection. It is characterized by progressive vitritis. The main measure of prevention is the use of povidone-iodine 5% antiseptic to clean the patient's eyes preoperatively.

FEATURES

Progressive vitritis (blurred vision, floaters), pain, hypopyon and corneal haze.

MANAGEMENT

Intravitreal antibiotics or pars plana vitrectomy. In acute endophthalmitis, the Early Vitrectomy Study Group found that early vitrectomy is only beneficial in patients with light perception-only vision (2).

11.6.1.1 ACUTE ENDOPHTHALMITIS

- Usually occurs within the first week of surgery.
- This is due to the patient's own periocular flora. The main causative organism is *Staphylococcus epidermidis.*

11.6.1.2 DELAYED ENDOPHTHALMITIS

- Onset varies from 6 weeks to several months.
- Main causative organism is *Propionibacterium acnes.*

11.6.1.3 OTHER CAUSES OF ENDOPHTHALMITIS

- Post-trauma: *Staphylococcus* or *Bacillus cereus* (has the worst prognosis).
- Fungal (*Candida*): Occurs in immunocompromised patients. Most common cause of endogenous endophthalmitis.

11.6.2 Posterior capsular opacification

This is the most common complication of late cataract surgery. The posterior capsule opacifies due to posterior migration of lens epithelial cells.

FEATURES

- Gradual loss of vision and glare; patients often think their cataracts have recurred.
- Elschnig pearls: Grape-like collection of swollen lens epithelial cells.
- Sommering rings: White annular proliferation of residual cells.

MANAGEMENT

- Capsulotomy with Nd:YAG laser.

11.7 CONGENITAL CATARACTS

OVERVIEW

- Bilateral cataracts comprise two-thirds of cases, AD in inheritance.
- Unilateral cataracts are usually sporadic in inheritance.

SECONDARY CAUSES OF CONGENITAL CATARACTS

1. Galactosaemia
   - AR condition due to absence of galactose-1-phosphate uridyltransferase.
   - Features: Infant presenting with liver dysfunction, failure to thrive and oil-droplet cataract.
   - Investigation: Stool for reducing substances.

- Management: Dietary restriction of lactose and galactose.
2. Lowe syndrome
   - XLR condition due to an abnormality in amino acid metabolism.
   - Features: Seizures, cataracts, posterior lenticonus and congenital glaucoma.
3. Fabry disease
   - Spoke-shaped posterior cataracts and corneal verticillata.
4. Mannosidosis
   - AR condition due to deficiency in alpha mannosidase.
   - Spoke-shaped posterior cataracts.
5. Down syndrome (trisomy 21)
   - Single palmar crease, low set ears, large tongue, epicanthal folds and blue dot cataract.
6. TORCH intrauterine infections
   - Toxoplasmosis, other (VZV, syphilis, parvovirus B19), rubella, CMV, HSV.

MANAGEMENT

- Observation, for small, <3 mm diameter, partial dense cataracts.
- In unilateral cases, part-time occlusion or pharmacological mydriasis of the good eye can be helpful to avoid amblyopia. These interventions are useful in delaying the need for cataract surgery until the eye growth becomes stable.
- Surgery: Involves pars plana lensectomy, posterior capsule capsulorhexis and anterior vitrectomy where appropriate. In addition to correction of refractive errors.
- A bilateral dense cataract requires surgical treatment within 8–10 weeks.
- A unilateral dense cataract requires surgical treatment within 6 weeks due to a higher risk of amblyopia.
- Postoperative complications
   - PCO: A dangerous complication, as it can lead to amblyopia.
   - Secondary glaucoma: Open-angle glaucoma can occur years after surgery. Angle closure may occur immediately postop. Incidence is higher if surgical treatment was performed within the first month of life.
   - Endophthalmitis.
   - Retinal detachment.

11.8 LENTICONUS

- Anterior lenticonus: Bilateral thinning of the anterior capsule with anterior lens protrusion into the anterior chamber. Associated with Alport syndrome (type IV collagen mutation disorder).

- Posterior lenticonus: Deformity in the posterior surface of the lens that is usually unilateral. Associated with congenital cataract. Associated with Lowe syndrome.

11.9 ECTOPIA LENTIS

Ectopia lentis refers to the dislocation/displacement of the lens from its normal position. The most common cause is trauma. However, it can be associated with ocular or systemic diseases.

11.9.1 Ocular causes

- Simple (familial) ectopia lentis
  - Occurs congenitally or later in life
  - Inheritance: AD or AR
  - Bilateral symmetric lens dislocation superotemporally
- Pseudoexfoliation syndrome
- Hypermature cataracts
- High myopia

11.9.2 Systemic causes

MARFAN SYNDROME

- Most common inherited cause of ectopia lentis.
- Inheritance: AD due to mutations of fibrillin-1 gene on chromosome 15 (FBN1 gene).
- Bilateral superotemporal lens dislocation is typical. Accommodation is not affected because zonules are intact. Ectopia lentis is the most common ocular feature.
- Systemic features
  - Tall stature, typically with dolichostenomelia (unusually long limbs)
  - Mitral prolapse, aortic aneurysm, regurgitation and dissection
  - Kyphoscoliosis

HOMOCYSTINURIA

- The second most common inherited cause of ectopia lentis.
- Inheritance: AR due to cystathionine beta-synthase deficiency.
- Bilateral inferonasal lens dislocation is typical.
- Systemic features
  - Coarse blond hair
  - Malar flush
  - Blue irides
  - Intellectual disability

REFERENCES

1. National Institute for Health and Care Excellence. Cataracts in Adults: Management. https://www.nice.org.uk/guidance/NG77. 2017.
2. Endophthalmitis Vitrectomy Study Group. Results of the Endophthalmitis Vitrectomy Study. A randomized trial of immediate vitrectomy and of intravenous antibiotics for the treatment of postoperative bacterial endophthalmitis. *Arch Ophthalmol.* 1995;113:1479–96.

12

Glaucoma

OMAR KOULI, RIZWAN MALIK AND STEWART GILLAN

12.1 ANATOMY AND PHYSIOLOGY

To understand glaucoma, one must first understand the physiology of the aqueous outflow and the relevant anatomy of the iridocorneal angle and optic nerve head.

12.1.1 Aqueous humour production

The ciliary body is made from the pars plicata anteriorly and pars plana posteriorly.

- The aqueous humour is formed by the ciliary processes in the pars plicata.
- There are three mechanisms of secretion:
  - Diffusion: Due to a concentration gradient.
  - Ultrafiltration: Pressure gradient between oncotic and hydrostatic pressures (capillary versus intraocular pressures).
  - Active ($\sim$80%): Active transport is mediated by transmembrane aquaporin activated by Na^+/K^+ ATPase enzyme and carbonic anhydrase enzyme.
- Control of aqueous secretion is controlled by the sympathetic (adrenergic innervation) system. β_2 receptor stimulation increases aqueous secretion; however, α_2 receptor stimulation decreases aqueous secretion.

12.1.2 Aqueous humour function and composition

- Function: Supplies essential nutrients for the cornea and lens.
- It fills the anterior chamber (volume of 0.25 mL; tends to become shallower with age and in people with hypermetropia) and posterior chamber (smaller than the anterior chamber).
- Composition
  - Water constitutes >99% of normal aqueous humour.
  - Lower concentrations of protein and glucose than plasma.
  - Higher concentrations of ascorbic acid, chloride and lactate than plasma.
  - Similar concentration of sodium to plasma.

12.1.3 Aqueous outflow routes

Aqueous humour travels through the posterior chamber into the anterior chamber. From there, aqueous humour can take one of two routes:

- Trabecular outflow ($\sim$70%): The conventional aqueous route in the eye going through the trabecular meshwork (TM) and Schlemm's canal to the episcleral veins.
- Uveoscleral outflow: Aqueous humour passes through the ciliary muscle to the suprachoroidal space and is eventually drained by choroidal veins, emissary canals of the sclera (vortex veins) or veins of the ciliary body.

12.1.4 Trabecular meshwork and Schlemm's canal

The TM consists of three parts:

- Uveal meshwork (innermost): Contains relatively large holes.
- Corneoscleral meshwork: Contains smaller holes, accounting for greater resistance.
- Juxtacanalicular meshwork (outermost): Connects the trabecular meshwork with the Schlemm canals. It contains narrow intercellular spaces, thus supplying the major part of the normal aqueous outflow resistance.

Schlemm's canal is an endothelial-lined oval canal situated circumferentially in the scleral sulcus. It contains holes for collector channels which terminate in the episcleral veins.

12.1.5 Optic nerve

NEURORETINAL RIM

- Refers to the area of the optic disc, between the margins of the central cup and the disc, containing retinal neuronal cells.
- The rim is thickest *Inferiorly*, followed by *Superiorly*, *Nasally* and *Temporally* (the 'ISNT rule').
- During glaucomatous changes, thinning of this neuroretinal rim occurs.

CUP TO DISC (C/D) RATIO

- Defined as the vertical diameter of the optic cup divided by the vertical diameter of the optic disc.
- The normal C/D ratio is 0.3. Some individuals may have physiological cupping of 0.6 or 0.7 without glaucomatous changes.

12.1.6 Trabeculectomy

- Trabeculectomy is an IOP-lowering surgical technique which involves the creation of a fistula for aqueous outflow from the anterior chamber to the sub-Tenon space, creating a bleb.
- Adjunctive use of antimetabolites may be used to slow the healing process in order to prevent bleb failure. Such antimetabolites are:
  - 5-fluorouracil (5-FU): A pyrimidine analogue which inhibits fibroblasts by blocking DNA synthesis.
  - Mitomycin C: An alkylating agent which also inhibits fibroblasts.

12.2 OCULAR HYPERTENSION

Ocular hypertension (OHT) is defined as raised IOP (>21 mmHg) without glaucomatous damage.

The Ocular Hypertension Treatment Study (OHTS) found that 9.5% of untreated patients with OHT converted to open-angle glaucoma in 5 years. However, with a 20% reduction of IOP (treated group) the 5-year risk conversion dropped to 4.4% (1). Risk factors for conversion, according to the OHTS, are:

- Older age.
- Higher IOP.
- Large cup/disc ratio.
- A thinner CCT: Patients with relatively thin central corneal thickness (CCT) (≤555 μm) had 3.4 times higher risk of conversion than patients with CCT >588 μm.
- Other risk factors that might contribute (not significant on multivariate analysis): African American origin, males and heart disease.

MANAGEMENT

- Regular monitoring.
- Medical treatment is indicated in cases with persistent IOP >30 mmHg or with high-risk profile patients.

12.3 PRIMARY OPEN-ANGLE GLAUCOMA

Primary open-angle glaucoma (POAG) is a chronic disorder characterized by glaucomatous visual field defects due to optic nerve damage. MYOC and OPTN gene mutations have the potential to cause POAG.

FEATURES

- Open anterior chamber angle
- High C/D ratio and thinning of the neuroretinal rim (Figure 12.1)
- Raised IOP (>21 mmHg)
- Glaucomatous VF defects

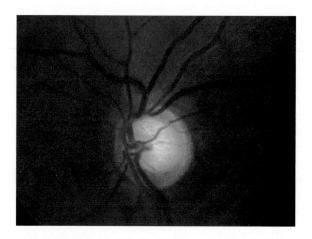

Figure 12.1 High C/D ratio.

INVESTIGATIONS

- Fundoscopy: Evaluate the optic disc.
- Gonioscopy: Assessment of angle.
- Pachymetry: Measure CCT.
- Perimetry: Visual field testing.

MANAGEMENT

- Topical IOP-lowering agents, such as prostaglandin analogues or beta-blockers.
- Laser trabeculoplasty.
- Trabeculectomy if failure of other treatments.

12.4 NORMAL-TENSION GLAUCOMA

Normal-tension glaucoma (NTG) is considered a form of POAG with a persistently normal IOP ($\leq$21 mmHg). Investigation and management are similar to POAG. Although the IOP in NTG is not elevated, the Collaborative Normal-Tension Glaucoma Study Group (2) showed that reducing IOP by 30% reduced the risk of progression of NTG (12% risk of progression in the treated group vs 35% in the untreated group in a 5-year follow-up).

RISK FACTORS

- Age: Commonly older than patients with POAG.
- Race: East Asian (e.g. Japanese).
- CCT: Commonly lower than patients with POAG.
- Systemic vascular disease: Conditions such as Raynaud phenomenon, migraines and systemic hypotension (use beta-blockers carefully due to their effect on blood pressure) are more associated with NTG rather than POAG.

FEATURES

Similar to POAG; however, notable differences:

- Optic nerve head can be larger in patients with NTG.
- Flame-shaped haemorrhages on optic nerve rim are more common in NTG.

12.5 PRIMARY ANGLE-CLOSURE GLAUCOMA

In primary angle-closure glaucoma (PACG), 'angle closure' refers to occlusion of the TM, causing obstruction of aqueous flow with the potential of causing a rise in IOP and optic nerve damage.

PACS VERSUS PAC VERSUS PACG

- Primary angle closure suspect (PACS): A narrow angle in which the peripheral iris is almost touching the TM. No peripheral anterior synechiae (PAS) present (PAS refers to the adherence of the peripheral iris anteriorly in the anterior chamber).
- Primary angle closure (PAC): PAS + elevated IOP. However, no glaucomatous optic nerve changes.
- Primary angle closure glaucoma (PACG): PAS + elevated IOP + glaucomatous changes and VF defects.

RISK FACTORS

- Increasing age
- East Asian race
- Hypermetropia
- Family history
- Short axial length of the eye

PATHOPHYSIOLOGY

- Relative pupillary block
  - Represents the majority of angle closure cases.
  - Failure of the normal aqueous flow through the pupil causes an increase in pressure difference between the posterior and anterior chambers. This results in the anterior bowing of the peripheral iris leading to angle closure.
  - Risk is highest in a mid-dilated pupil due to maximum contact between iris and lens at this level.
- Plateau iris configuration (non-pupillary block): Important pathophysiological mechanism in the East Asian descents. Characterized by a flat iris, normal anterior chamber depth and anteriorly positioned ciliary processes which displaces the iris base leading to a narrow/closed angle.

FEATURES

- Sudden onset headache, vomiting, haloes and blurring or transient visual loss. Symptoms are exacerbated by watching TV in a dark room, pharmacological mydriasis or reading.
- Fixed mid-dilated pupil, corneal oedema, conjunctival hyperaemia and highly raised IOP.
- Resolved acute attack: Descemet membrane folds, low IOP and glaukomflecken.

MANAGEMENT

- Acute: Supine position, systemic acetazolamide, topical beta-blockers ± alpha-2 agonists ± topical prednisolone.
- Bilateral peripheral Nd: YAG laser iridotomies to be performed after resolution of acute attack.
- Cataract extraction has shown to be effective in lowering IOP in both acute and chronic stages of the disease.

12.6 NEOVASCULAR GLAUCOMA (NVG)

Neovascular glaucoma (NVG) is a cause of either secondary open- or closed-angle glaucoma. NVG occurs due to proliferation of fibrovascular tissue in the anterior angle and results from rubeosis iridis (Figure 12.2).

CAUSES

- Ischaemic central retinal vein occlusion (CRVO) (NVG usually occurs about 3 months after onset of CRVO '100-day glaucoma').
- Central retinal artery occlusion (CRAO).
- Diabetes mellitus.
- Ocular ischaemic syndrome.
- Retinal detachment.

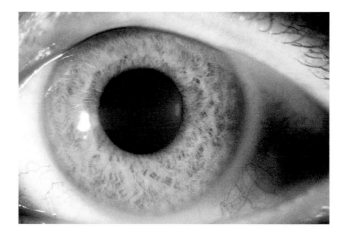

Figure 12.2 Iris neovascularisation (rubeosis iridis).

PATHOPHYSIOLOGY

- Retinal ischaemia.
- Hypoxia to the retina cells.
- Release of angiogenic factors (VEGF and IL-6).
- The result is neovascularization of the anterior segment (iris and iridocorneal angle) with subsequent overlying fibrovascular membrane formation.

FEATURES

- New radially orientated vessels on iris surface and pupillary margins.
- PAS and posterior synechiae can form.
- Corneal oedema.
- Elevated IOP with open angle at the beginning but progression will lead to fibrovascular tissue proliferation leading to PAS formation and angle closure.

INVESTIGATIONS

- Establish the cause of retinal ischaemia.

MANAGEMENT

- PRP ± intravitreal anti-VEGF injections to reduce neovascularisation.
- Medical treatment
  - Similar to POAG.
  - Avoid miotic agents, as they can worsen synechial angle closure.
  - Use prostaglandin analogues carefully because they may exacerbate ocular inflammation.
  - Osmotic agents can be used for corneal oedema.
- Surgery (if medical treatment fails)
  - If *good* visual prognosis = glaucoma drainage device (tube).

- If *bad* visual potential = cyclodiode laser (destruction of the ciliary body epithelium leading to reduction of aqueous humour secretion).
- Trabeculectomy can often result in bleb failure due to scarring.

12.7 PIGMENT DISPERSION SYNDROME

An AD-inherited cause of secondary open-angle glaucoma, characterized by excessive 'shedding' of pigmented material of the iris deposited throughout the anterior segment. It is more common in myopic males.

FEATURES

Blurred vision and haloes on exertion. The following signs may be seen:

- Mid-peripheral spoke-like defects of the iris on transillumination (Figure 12.3).
- Increased IOP and glaucomatous damage.
- Vertical oval-shaped pigments on the corneal endothelium (Krukenberg spindles).
- TM pigmentation.
- Sampaolesi line may be present (a band of pigmented anterior to the Schwalbe line on gonioscopy).
- Concave peripheral iris.

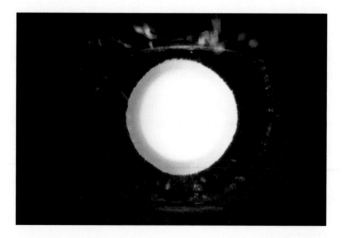

Figure 12.3 Mid-peripheral spoke-like transillumination defects in pigment dispersion.

MANAGEMENT

- Avoid extraneous exercise.
- Medical treatment is similar to POAG. Prostaglandin analogues are generally the preferred medical treatment for patients, although other topical medications may be used.

- Pilocarpine has shown to be a prophylactic measure to prevent exercise-induced elevation of IOP. However, the use of miotics (pilocarpine) can induce myopia and have risk of retinal detachment.
- Laser trabeculoplasty.
- Trabeculectomy.

12.8 PSEUDOEXFOLIATION SYNDROME

This is a cause of secondary open-angle glaucoma in which grey-white fibrillar deposits block the anterior chamber angle. Associated with mutation in the LOXL1 (enzyme that contributes to elastin formation). More likely to present in Scandinavians, females and age >50. Investigations and treatment similar to POAG.

ASSOCIATIONS
- Hearing loss
- Alzheimer disease
- High plasma homocysteine levels
- Low folate intake

FEATURES
- Increased IOP and glaucomatous damage.
- Flaky white deposits on the anterior lens capsule.
- Sampaolesi line.
- Peripupillary defect on transillumination slit lamp.

12.9 POSNER-SCHLOSSMAN SYNDROME

A rare disorder characterized by recurrent unilateral acute attacks of IOP elevation and may cause secondary open-angle glaucoma (uncommon, only if repeated attacks). More likely in middle-aged patients. Associated with CMV or *Helicobacter pylori* infection and HLA-BW5.

FEATURES
- Discomfort, haloes and blurred vision.
- Anterior chamber inflammation.
- Mydriasis.

TREATMENT
- Topical steroids and IOP-lowering agents.

12.10 PHACOLYTIC GLAUCOMA

A secondary open-angle glaucoma caused by trabecular obstruction due to leakage of lens protein from a hypermature cataract.

FEATURES

- Painful red eye with photophobia and decreased vision.
- Corneal oedema, mature cataract and white particles may be seen in the anterior chamber due to an inflammatory response against the lens protein present in the anterior chamber.

TREATMENT

- Topical or systemic IOP-lowering agents.
- Definitive treatment: cataract extraction.

12.11 PHACOMORPHIC GLAUCOMA

An acute secondary angle-closure glaucoma due to a swelling of a cataractous lens potentiating a pupillary block. Presentation is similar to acute PACG.

TREATMENT

- IOP reduction: Same as acute PACG (avoid miotics: can potentiate pupillary block).
- Definitive treatment: Cataract extraction.

12.12 RED CELL GLAUCOMA

A hyphema (collection of blood inside the anterior chamber) can form, usually following blunt trauma to the eye, which leads to blockage of the TM leading to raised IOP and secondary open angle glaucoma. A secondary bleed may occur 3–7 days post initial injury.

12.13 GHOST CELL GLAUCOMA

A type of secondary open-angle glaucoma occurring 2–4 weeks after a vitreous haemorrhage due to TM obstruction with red blood cells.

12.14 ANGLE RECESSION GLAUCOMA

A cause of chronic secondary open-angle glaucoma due to ciliary body rupture caused by blunt trauma. Gonioscopy shows irregular widening of the ciliary body face. The risk of glaucoma occurring is about 10% after 10 years following the traumatic incident.

12.15 STURGE-WEBER SYNDROME

A congenital neuro-oculocutaneous disorder that can cause secondary open-angle glaucoma.

PATHOPHYSIOLOGY OF GLAUCOMA

Anterior chamber angle malformation (causes early-onset glaucoma during the first year of life) or increased episcleral venous pressure (causes later-onset glaucoma).

FEATURES

- Cutaneous: Port wine stain, typically along CNV_1 and CNV_2.
- Neurological: Seizures and learning disability.
- Ocular: Choroidal haemangiomas and glaucoma ipsilateral to the cutaneous lesion.

TREATMENT

- Early-onset glaucoma: Goniotomy or trabeculotomy or combined trabeculotomy-trabeculectomy.
- Late-onset glaucoma: Medical therapy first, then trabeculectomy if medical therapy fails.

12.16 PRIMARY CONGENITAL GLAUCOMA

Primary congenital glaucoma (PCG) is a rare bilateral (two-thirds of patients) condition due to malformation of the anterior chamber angle that occurs in the first year of life.

EPIDEMIOLOGY

- More common in boys.
- Mostly sporadic, however, can be AR.
- Prevalence higher in patients with CYP_1B_1 gene.

FEATURES

- Photophobia, epiphora and blepharospasm.
- Corneal oedema.
- Large corneal diameter (>12 mm).
- Buphthalmos: Large eyes due to elevated IOP.
- Haab striae: Healed breaks in Descemet's membrane due to corneal oedema. Best seen on retroillumination.

INVESTIGATIONS

- IOP measurement (normal IOP in newborns is 10–12 mmHg).
- Optic disc evaluation for cupping: Look for asymmetry or a ratio of >0.3.
- Corneal diameter measurement (normal range is 9.5–10.5 mm in newborns).

MANAGEMENT

- Angle surgery: Goniotomy if the cornea is clear. If the cornea is cloudy, then trabeculotomy can be tried.

REFERENCES

1. Gordon MO, Beiser JA, Brandt JD et al. The Ocular Hypertension Treatment Study: Baseline factors that predict the onset of primary open-angle glaucoma. *Arch Ophthalmol.* 2002;120(6):714–20.
2. Collaborative Normal-Tension Glaucoma Study Group. Comparison of glaucomatous progression between untreated patients with normal-tension glaucoma and patients with therapeutically reduced intraocular pressures. *Am J Ophthalmol.* 1998;126(4):487–97.

13

Uveitis

MOSTAFA KHALIL, OMAR KOULI AND OBAID KOUSHA

13.1 ANATOMY

The uvea consists of the iris, ciliary body and choroid.

13.1.1 The iris

The iris is the most anterior part of the uvea containing muscles to allow pupillary size changes. The iris consists of two structures: the stroma and the posterior pigmented layer.

STROMA

The stroma is composed of many cells including melanocytes (pigmented cells) that gives the iris its colour. It has two zones:

1. The *pupillary zone* extends from the pupillary edge to the collarette (thickest part of the iris that separates the two zones). The sphincter pupillae is located here. It is a smooth muscle responsible for pupillary constriction with parasympathetic innervation (CNIII) via short ciliary nerves.
2. The *ciliary zone* extends from the collarette to the origin of the iris at the ciliary body. The dilator pupillae is located here. It is a smooth muscle responsible for pupillary dilatation with sympathetic innervation via long ciliary nerves.

POSTERIOR PIGMENTED LAYER

A pigmented epithelial layer found at the posterior iris surface that is continuous with the neurosensory retina posteriorly.

13.1.2 Ciliary body

The ciliary body consists of three layers: stroma (connective tissue where the vascular supply is found), muscle (parasympathetic innervation via CNIII) and epithelium. The blood supply to the ciliary body is via the anterior and long posterior ciliary arteries. The ciliary body is divided into two parts: pars plana and pars plicata.

1. Pars plana: Avascular. Lies between the ora serrata and ciliary processes of the pars plicata. Functionless, often used as a site for intravitreal injections or vitreous removal (pars plana vitrectomy).
2. Pars plicata: Highly vascularized. Forms attachments for the lens zonules. Functions include aqueous humour formation, lens accommodation and aqueous drainage via uveoscleral outflow.

13.1.3 Choroid

The choroid is the posterior component of the uveal tract. It lies between the sclera externally and retinal pigmented epithelium (RPE) internally. Its function is to provide nutrients to the outer third of the retina. It consists of Bruch's membrane and a vascular layer.

1. Bruch's membrane: The innermost layer before the RPE. It is a highly homogenous structure consisting of five layers measuring less than 4 micrometres. The function is not clear; however, it may play a role in fluid transport from the choroid to the retina and is permeable to small molecules (e.g. fluorescein).
2. Vascular layer: Consists of three layers: choriocapillaries which are external to the Bruch membrane, a medium-sized vessel layer and a large vessel layer. The choroid is perfused via two long posterior ciliary arteries, the short posterior ciliary artery and anterior ciliary artery.

13.2 UVEITIS

Uveitis is defined as inflammation of the uveal tract ± inflammation of the surrounding structures (e.g. retina, vitreous or anterior chamber). It is split into anterior, intermediate and posterior uveitis or pan-uveitis (whole uveal tract inflammation).

13.2.1 Anterior uveitis

Inflammation of the iris ± pars plicata (anterior ciliary body). *Synonym*: iritis.

Anterior uveitis can be classified into acute/chronic (chronic if >3 months) or granulomatous/nongranulomatous.

GRANULOMATOUS VERSUS NONGRANULOMATOUS

Keratic precipitates (KPs) which are white blood cells on the posterior endothelial layer of the cornea. Granulomatous is defined by mutton fat KPs whereas nongranulomatous is defined with stellate KPs.

AETIOLOGY
- Idiopathic (50%).
- HLA-B27-associated conditions (psoriasis, reactive arthritis, inflammatory bowel disease and ankylosing spondylitis).
- Inflammatory: Sarcoidosis, Behçet syndrome, systemic lupus erythematosus, juvenile idiopathic arthritis, multiple sclerosis (MS), Fuchs' heterochromic cyclitis, tubulointerstitial nephritis, Posner-Schlossman syndrome.
- Infectious: Tuberculosis (TB), Lyme disease, syphilis, varicella zoster virus (VZV).

FEATURES

Painful red eye, blurred vision and photophobia. Possible findings on examination:

- Irregular miosed pupil: Due to inflammation of the sphincter pupillae of the iris. May predispose to posterior synechiae (adhesion between the iris and lens capsule).

- Anterior chamber cells: Due to inflammation of the ciliary body which produces aqueous humour.
- KP: Stellate or mutton fat depending on aetiology.
- Hypopyon: White cells in the anterior chamber.
- Iris atrophy and nodules: More common in chronic cases.
- Complications: Cystoid macular oedema (CMO) and cataracts.

MANAGEMENT

- Investigate as appropriate based on clinical findings. For example, measuring calcium and serum ACE if sarcoidosis is suspected.
- Potent topical steroid and cyclopentolate to dilate the pupil.

13.2.2 Intermediate uveitis

Inflammation of the posterior ciliary body (pars plana) and vitreous. *Synonym*: pars planitis.

AETIOLOGY

- Idiopathic.
- Inflammatory: Sarcoidosis, MS, inflammatory bowel disease (ulcerative colitis and Crohn disease).
- Infectious: Lyme disease.

FEATURES

Patients often present with blurred vision and floaters. There is no pain or red eye. Examination findings:

- Snowballs: White focal inflammatory cells and exudates. Most commonly in the inferior vitreous.
- Snowbanking: Whitish exudates in the ora serrata, typically inferiorly, that may extend into the pars plana. It can be viewed via an indirect ophthalmoscope with scleral depression.
- Peripheral periphlebitis (especially in MS).

COMPLICATIONS

- CMO
- Optic disc swelling
- Band keratopathy
- Glaucoma
- Cataracts: From steroid use

13.2.3 Posterior uveitis

Inflammation of the choroid ± retina. *Synonym*: chorioretinitis.

AETIOLOGY

- Idiopathic.
- Inflammatory: Sympathetic ophthalmia, Vogt-Koyanagi-Harada (VKH) syndrome, birdshot choroidopathy, sarcoidosis, Behçet syndrome.
- Infectious: Toxoplasmosis, onchocerciasis, toxocariasis, syphilis, TB, VZV, herpes simplex virus (HSV), cytomegalovirus (CMV).

13.3 SARCOIDOSIS

Inflammatory multisystem disorder characterized by noncaseating granulomas. Histopathology includes multinucleated giant cells of Langerhans type and Schaumann bodies. More common in African-Caribbean patients.

EXTRAOCULAR FEATURES

- Bilateral hilar lymphadenopathy
- Erythema nodosum
- Bilateral CNVII palsy
- Bilateral parotid enlargement

OCULAR FEATURES

Anterior, intermediate, posterior or pan-uveitis. Unilateral or bilateral.
- Anterior uveitis: Mutton fat KPs and iris nodules.
- Intermediate uveitis with snowbanking and snowballs.
- Posterior uveitis
  - CMO
  - Candle wax: Patchy periphlebitis
  - Choroiditis
  - Periretinal granuloma (Lander sign): Specific to sarcoidosis only and not seen in TB

DIAGNOSIS

- High serum ACE, calcium levels
- Chest x-ray and spirometry

13.4 TUBERCULOSIS

Infection by *Mycobacterium tuberculosis* (acid-fast bacilli seen on Ziehl-Neelsen stain) causing caseating granulomas in the body. More common in patients from India. Multiple organs can be affected.

EXTRAOCULAR FEATURES

- Night sweats
- Weight loss
- Fevers and rigors
- Haemoptysis

OCULAR FEATURES

- Conjunctivitis, scleritis or keratitis.
- Anterior uveitis: Mutton fat KPs and iris nodules.
- Posterior uveitis
  - Vitritis
  - Retinal vasculitis with vascular occlusions can occur
  - Choroiditis and choroidal granuloma
  - CMO
- Lacrimal gland: Dacryoadenitis.

13.5 SYMPATHETIC OPHTHALMIA

Bilateral T-cell-mediated granulomatous pan-uveitis which occurs days or years following ocular surgery or trauma. It is associated with HLA-DR4 and HLA-A11.

FEATURES

- Pain: Due to anterior uveitis and/or optic neuritis.
- Granulomatous anterior uveitis.
- Vitritis.
- Choroidal infiltrates.
- Dalen-Fuchs' nodules: Pigmented epithelioid cells between RPE and Bruch membrane.

MANAGEMENT

- Steroids.
- Enoculation: Prevents fellow eye from developing sympathetic ophthalmia – best option for eyes that are blind.

13.6 VOGT-KOYANAGI-HARADA SYNDROME

Bilateral granulomatous pan-uveitis associated with multisystem inflammation. The condition is more common in the Japanese population. May be due to T-cell response against melanocytes, melanin and the RPE. Associated with HLA-DR4 and HLA-B22. This condition is distinct from sympathetic ophthalmia in that there is a lack of trauma and there are extraocular signs.

FEATURES

- Bilateral pan-uveitis.
- Dalen-Fuchs' nodules.
- Depigmented limbus (Sugiura sign) and depigmented fundus ('sunset glow' appearance).
- Exudative retinal detachment.
- Systemic: Alopecia, vitiligo, sensorineural hearing loss and meningitis.

MANAGEMENT

- Systemic steroids

13.7 BIRDSHOT CHOROIDOPATHY

Chronic and bilateral posterior uveitis with characteristic hypopigmented fundus lesions. Strong association with HLA-A29. Predominantly affects middle-aged females.

FEATURES

Insidious impairment of central vision with flashes, floaters and nyctalopia. Signs include:

- Moderate vitritis (no snowbanking/snowballs).
- Bilateral oval cream-coloured ill-defined lesions in posterior pole and mid-periphery.

INVESTIGATIONS

- FA: Early hypofluorescence with late hyperfluorescence.
- ERG: Prolonged 30 Hz flicker times.

13.8 FUCHS' HETEROCHROMIC CYCLITIS

Nongranulomatous unilateral disorder causing a chronic anterior uveitis, posterior subcapsular cataract and a chronic open-angle glaucoma.

FEATURES

- Chronic anterior uveitis: White eye, stellate KPs, anterior chamber flare.
- Iris atrophy and heterochromia (affected iris is hypochromic).
- Posterior subcapsular cataract: dVa and glare.
- Glaucoma.

13.9 TUBULOINTERSTITIAL NEPHRITIS AND UVEITIS

Bilateral granulomatous anterior uveitis that occurs in patients with tubulointerstitial nephritis (TIN). Commonly presents in female teenagers.

FEATURES

Renal disease occurs before ocular disease. Patients present with fever, malaise, flank pain, proteinuria and anaemia (renal disease). Anterior uveitis presents with painful red eye and photophobia, miosed pupil with anterior chamber flare and stellate KPs. Increased beta-2 microglobinuria in the urine is seen.

13.10 JUVENILE IDIOPATHIC ARTHRITIS

The most common rheumatological disease in children and also the most common cause of anterior uveitis in children. The aetiology is unknown; however, there is an association with HLA-DR5. This condition is more common in females.

FEATURES

- Arthritis: Most common type that is seen is oligoarthritis (≤4 joints affected). Must be present for 6 weeks.
- Ophthalmic: Chronic and nongranulomatous anterior uveitis, cataract and band keratopathy.
- Spiking fevers (lasting 2 weeks) and rashes are also commonly seen.

MANAGEMENT

- ANA is usually positive. Steroids are the mainstay treatment.

13.11 REITER SYNDROME

Infectious cause of arthritis and conjunctivitis with an immunological component (HLA-B27).

AETIOLOGY

Non-gonococcal infections:

- GU: Chlamydia
- GI: Shigella, Salmonella, Yersinia

FEATURES

- Triad: Conjunctivitis, urethritis, arthritis
- Less commonly: Iritis, keratitis, prostatitis, keratoderma blennorrhagica

13.12 BEHÇET DISEASE

Rare multisystem vasculitis that occurs more commonly in those of Turkish descent. Associated with HLA-B51.

FEATURES

- Recurrent oral and genital ulcers
- Erythema nodosum
- Anterior uveitis with pathogenomic mobile hypopyon
- Positive pathergy skin test: Skin lesions in response to minor trauma
- Pulmonary artery aneurysm (pathogenomic)

MANAGEMENT

- Steroid therapy and anti-TNF agents

13.13 KAWASAKI DISEASE

A medium-vessel vasculitis.

FEATURES

Suspect in any patient (usually children) with a fever lasting longer than 5 days that is not responsive to typical antipyretics such as paracetamol.

- Eyes
  - Bilateral conjunctival injection sparing the limbus
  - Bilateral anterior uveitis
- Mouth: Strawberry tongue
- Skin: Shedding rash of the extremities

MANAGEMENT

- Aspirin (only agent to reduce the fever)
- IV immunoglobulins

COMPLICATIONS

- Coronary artery aneurysm: All patients require an echocardiogram to exclude this complication.

13.14 ONCHOCERCIASIS

Caused by *Onchocerca volvulus*, with *Simulium* black fly being the vector. Endemic in Africa and South America. It is the second leading cause of infectious blindness in the world behind trachoma. Treated with ivermectin.

FEATURES

A maculopapular rash is often the first sign seen and precedes ocular features, which include:

- dVA.
- Sclerosing keratitis: Subepithelial punctate lesions (snowflake opacities).
- Anterior uveitis: Painful red eye with photophobia. Pearly shaped pupil (due to posterior synechiae; attachment of the iris to the lens, may predispose to glaucoma and increase IOP).
- Bilateral chorioretinitis with RPE atrophy.
- Optic neuritis and atrophy.
- Visualization of the nematode on slit lamp retroillumination.

13.15 TOXOCARIASIS

Commonly caused by *Toxocara cani*, with dogs being the definitive hosts.

FEATURES

Unilateral endophthalmitis in children aged 2–6:

- Progressive vitritis, grey-white exudates.
- Leukocoria, strabismus, visual loss.

- Anterior uveitis: Pain photophobia, etc.
- Pars planitis: Snowballs.

INVESTIGATIONS
- Absence of calcification on CT scan.
- Differentiates from retinoblastoma, another cause of leukocoria in that age group.

MANAGEMENT
- Corticosteroids play an important role.
- Surgery may be indicated.
- Limited role for antihelmintics such as thiabendazole.

13.16 AIDS-RELATED CONDITIONS

Toxoplasmosis, presumed ocular histoplasmosis syndrome (POHS), CMV retinitis, and progressive outer retinal necrosis (PORN) are all AIDS-related conditions and are discussed below. Acute retinal necrosis (ARN) is not associated with AIDS but will also be discussed to compare with PORN.

13.17 TOXOPLASMOSIS

Caused by the parasite *Toxoplasma gondii*, from cats. This condition occurs in patients with AIDS, specifically with CD4+ counts <200.

FEATURES
- Congenital toxoplasmosis
  - Triad: Hydrocephalus, intraretinal calcification and chorioretinitis.
  - Sabin Fieldman test positive.
  - Management: Pyrimethamine (folic acid antagonist).
- Acquired toxoplasmosis
  - White lesion of retinitis with an associated pigmented scar (Figure 13.1).

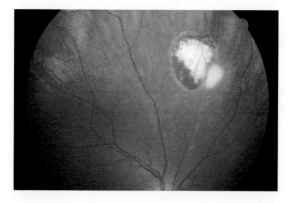

Figure 13.1 Toxoplasmosis.

- Focal retinitis with overlying vitritis ('headlight in the fog').
- 'Spillover' anterior uveitis: Due to vitreous spilling in anterior chamber.
- Management: Pyrimethamine + sulfadiazine + corticosteroid.

13.18 PRESUMED OCULAR HISTOPLASMOSIS SYNDROME

This clinical presentation occurs due to *Histoplasma capsulatum* (dimorphic fungi). Associated with HLA-B7 and HLA-DR2. Famously occurs in Ohio, Mississippi, and St Lawrence River valleys. More common in patients with AIDS.

FEATURES

- Patient usually presents with loss of vision.
- Examination findings (triad)
    - Multiple white atrophic punched-out chorioretinal scars
    - Peripapillary atrophy
    - Absent vitritis

COMPLICATIONS

- Choroidal neovascularization – late manifestation.
- Exudative macular detachment.

13.19 CYTOMEGALOVIRUS RETINITIS

A weak opportunistic infection that only occurs in AIDS patients when the CD4+ count is less than 50. This infection can present in the eye and cause full-thickness retinal inflammation with necrosis, retinal tears and detachments. Treatment is with IV ganciclovir.

FEATURES

- Rapid visual loss.
- Mainly posterior pole affected.
- Pizza pie/cottage cheese-with-ketchup appearance indicating prominent haemorrhages (Figure 13.2).
- Periphlebitis, frosted branch angiitis (vein and artery involvement).
- Mild-moderate vitritis.

13.20 PROGRESSIVE OUTER RETINAL NECROSIS

This is a devastating necrotizing retinitis caused by VZV in AIDS patients with a CD4+ count less than 50. Treatment is with IV ganciclovir.

FEATURES

- Very rapid visual loss.
- Multifocal yellow/white retinal infiltrates.

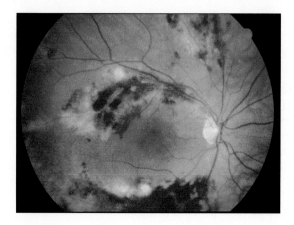

Figure 13.2 CMV retinitis.

- Rapidly conjugating white areas of peripheral retinal necrosis.
- Minimal vasculitis, absent vitritis.

13.21 ACUTE RETINAL NECROSIS

Devastating pan-uveitis *not* associated with AIDS. Treatment is with IV acyclovir.

AETIOLOGY
- VZV: Older patients
- HSV: Children

FEATURES
- Rapid loss of visual acuity; floaters, discomfort.
- Predominantly a peripheral disease of occlusive arteritis.
- Full-thickness peripheral retinal necrotising retinitis.
- Marked vitritis.

Medical retina

MOSTAFA KHALIL AND OBAID KOUSHA

14.1 ANATOMY AND PHYSIOLOGY

14.1.1 Vitreous

The vitreous is the largest cavity, 4.0–4.4 mL in adulthood, of the eye that contains viscoelastic gel made of mostly water. Besides water, the vitreous humour contains mainly hyaluronic acid and type II collagen.

14.1.2 Retina overview

The retina is the layer responsible for converting light energy into neural signals. It is derived embryologically from the diencephalon. The diencephalon gives rise to the optic vesicle and then the optic cup.

The retina is composed of two main parts:

- The outer retinal pigment epithelium (RPE) layer – From the outer optic cup of the diencephalon.
- The inner neurosensory retina (NSR) (composed of nine layers) – From the inner optic cup of the diencephalon.

There is therefore a weak connection between the RPE and the NSR, which is why retinal detachment occurs (the separation of the NSR from the RPE).

14.1.3 Neurosensory retina

The nine layers of the NSR, from inwards to outwards, are as follows:

1. Internal limiting membrane: Separates the retina from the vitreous.
2. Nerve fibre layer (NFL): Contains ganglion cell axons that come together to form the optic nerve. Presents in the macular area and travels nasally to the optic nerve directly through the papillomacular bundle.
3. Ganglion cell layer: Contains the cell bodies of the ganglion cells. Involved in transmitting visual information to the brain including the stimulus required for light pupillary response.
4. Inner plexiform layer: Synaptic layer between second and third order neurons.
5. Inner nuclear layer: Contains cell bodies of bipolar cells and cell bodies of Müller cells (principal glial cells of the retina).
6. Outer plexiform layer: Synaptic layer between photoreceptors and bipolar cells.
7. Outer nuclear layer: Contains cell bodies of rods and cones.
8. External limiting membrane (ELM): Connections between photoreceptors and Muller cells create the ELM.
9. Photoreceptor layer: Composed of rods and cones.

14.1.4 Retinal pigment epithelium

The retinal pigment epithelium (RPE) is composed of a single layer of cuboidal epithelial cells containing melanosomes and has many functions:

- Absorbs light and prevents the scattering of light within the eye.
- Replenishes the molecules needed for phototransduction.
- Contains a blood-retinal barrier, which provides a selectively permeable membrane to supply nutrients to the photoreceptors and maintain homeostasis. The blood-retinal barrier is maintained by the zonulae occludentes.
- Phagocytosis of photoreceptor outer segment membranes.
- Transport and storage of metabolites and vitamins.

14.1.5 Macula lutea

- The macula is a pigmented, rounded area at the posterior pole of the retina, located temporal to the optic disc.
- It contains several layers of ganglion cells in contrast to the peripheral retina, which contains only one layer.
- The fovea is a depression at the centre of the macula that contains only cones and represents the retina's highest visual acuity. The centre of the fovea is avascular and is dependent on the underlying choriocapillaris for blood supply via diffusion.

14.1.6 The photoreceptors

Table 14.1 explains the differences between rods and cons.

Table 14.1 Rods versus cones

	Rods	Cones
Quantity	120 million	6 million
Location	Highest density in the mid-peripheral retina (about 20° from point of fixation)	Highest density at the macula (especially the fovea)
Pigment	Rhodopsin	Iodopsin
Wavelength of maximum absorbance (nm)	498	Three types: Short (420), medium (534) and long (564) wavelength cones which are sensitive to blue, green and red light, respectively
Bipolar connection	One bipolar cell can receive stimuli from multiple rods	Forms a 1:1 ratio with bipolar cells
Function	Sensitive in dark-dim illumination	Sensitive to bright light
	Responsible for night and peripheral vision	Responsible for central and colour vision

14.1.7 Blood supply to the retina

- The outer third of retinal layers, including photoreceptors and RPE, are supplied by the short posterior ciliary artery (choroid).
- The inner two-thirds of retinal layers are supplied by the central retinal artery.
- Variation: In some patients, the inner layer of the macula may have a dual blood supply by the cilioretinal arteries (branch of the short posterior ciliary artery). When unaffected, central vision may be conserved in cases of central retinal artery occlusion (CRAO).

14.2 DIABETIC RETINOPATHY AND MACULOPATHY

Diabetic retinopathy (DR) is the most common microvascular complication of diabetes and is the most common cause of blindness in adults aged 35–65 in developed countries.

PATHOGENESIS

Hyperglycaemia causes increased retinal blood flow and damage to endothelial walls and pericytes. Endothelial dysfunction causes vascular permeability and hard exudate formation (lipoproteins in the outer plexiform layer).

- Pericyte damage predisposes to the formation of microaneurysms, which are leakages of blood from capillary walls and flame haemorrhages due to rupture of the capillary walls which track along the nerve fibre layer.
- Cotton wool spot formation: Axonal debris at margins of ischaemic infarcts.
- Neovascularization occurs through angiogenic factors such as vascular endothelial growth factor (VEGF) in response to ischaemia.
- Cystoid macular oedema (CMO): Most layers can be affected, particularly the outer plexiform layer.

RISK FACTORS

- Duration of diabetes: Most important risk factor.
- Poor diabetic control
  - For type 2 diabetics, a 37% reduction in progression rate of microvascular complications (e.g. retinopathy) can be achieved with 1% reduction in HbA1c (1).
  - For insulin-dependent diabetics, intensive glycaemic therapy showed a 76% reduction in progression of retinopathy when compared to the control group. Note, however, intensive diabetic control may transiently worsen retinopathy in the first few months (2).
- Pregnancy.
- Other factors: Smoking, hyperlipidaemia and hypertension (for type 2 diabetics, a tight blood pressure control with a mean of 144/82 mmHg caused a 37% reduction of microvascular complications [3]).

FEATURES

Most patients will be asymptomatic. However, causes of vision loss include:

- Gradual onset
    - Any type of diabetic retinopathy.
    - Diabetic macular oedema: Most common cause of visual impairment.
    - Cataract.
- Acute onset
    - Painless: Similar to vitreous haemorrhage or tractional retinal detachment (flashes and floaters may precede visual loss).
    - Painful: Similar to neovascular glaucoma (NVG) precipitated by rubeosis iridis.

CLASSIFICATION

DR can be classified according to the modified Airlie House classification developed by the Diabetic Retinopathy Study (4) and used by the Early Treatment Diabetic Retinopathy Study (ETDRS) (5) follows.

Nonproliferative DR

This can be further split into mild, moderate and severe based on the following clinical findings:

- *Mild*
    - At least one microaneurysm, intraretinal haemorrhages, exudates or cotton wool spots.
- *Moderate*
    - Intraretinal haemorrhages (in 1–3 quadrants) or mild intraretinal microvascular abnormality (IRMA-shunt vessels that arise to supply hypoperfused areas).
    - Venous beading (in 1 quadrant only).
- *Severe* (Figure 14.1)

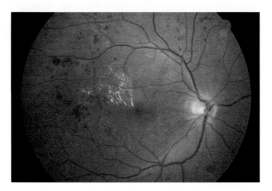

Figure 14.1 A nonproliferative severe diabetic retinopathy.

- Follows the 4-2-1 rule; one or more of:
    - Intraretinal haemorrhages in 4 quadrants
    - Venous beading $\geq$ 2 quadrants
    - Moderate IRMA $\geq$ 1 quadrant

Proliferative DR

This can be split into non-high risk, high risk and advanced.

- *Non-high risk*
    - Neovascularization on disc (NVD) or elsewhere (NVE) (Figure 14.2).

- *High risk*
    - Fulfils one of the following:
        - NV >1/3 disc area
        - NVD plus vitreous haemorrhage
        - NVE >1/2 disc area plus vitreous haemorrhage

- *Advanced*
    - Tractional RD

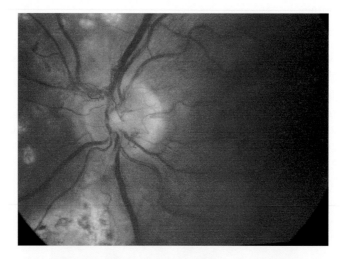

Figure 14.2 Neovascularization on the optic disc.

Diabetic maculopathy

Defined by the presence of diabetic macular oedema (DMO), classified as:

- Centre involving DMO *or*
- Extra-foveal DMO meeting clinically significant macular oedema (CSMO) defined by the ETDRS (5).

INVESTIGATIONS

- Optical coherence tomography (OCT) for assessing and monitoring DMO.
- Fluorescence angiography (FA) mainly used to assess for retinal ischaemia.

MANAGEMENT (6)

- Glycaemic and blood pressure control (use effective antihypertensives such as lisinopril).
- Nonproliferative DR
  - Monitoring in screening programmes or secondary care ranging from annual (for mild-moderate) to 4 monthly (severe).
  - Consider pan-retinal photocoagulation (PRP) for severe nonproliferative in elderly patients with type 2 diabetes or if poor attendance or prior to cataract surgery.
- Proliferative DR
  - Non-high risk: Regular routine review ± PRP.
  - High risk: PRP within 2 weeks. Treat DMO, if coexists, at the same time or before.
- Vitreous haemorrhage: Treat as high-risk PDR.
- Tractional RD or persistent vitreous haemorrhage: Pars plana vitrectomy.
- Maculopathy
  - Treated with intravitreal anti-VEGF (ranibizumab or aflibercept, note the latter has a higher molecular weight and is second line) if there is DMO on OCT and the vision is affected.
  - Consider using modified ETDRS laser if anti-VEGF is contraindicated (e.g. pregnancy).
- Diabetic retinopathy and cataract surgery: Treat CSMO and PDR or neovascularization of iris before cataract surgery. If there is no fundal view perform B scan ultrasound.

14.3 HYPERTENSIVE RETINOPATHY

Atherosclerotic changes and vasoconstriction of retinal arteries in response to chronic hypertension causes endothelial damage and can lead to retinopathy (see stages below). Chronic hypertensive retinopathy can include similar signs to diabetic retinopathy. Management is usually with BP control.

CLINICAL STAGES OF HYPERTENSIVE RETINOPATHY

1. Arteriolar narrowing.
2. Arteriovenous nipping (Figure 14.3) or atherosclerosis with thickening of retinal arterioles ('copper/silver wiring').
3. Stage 2 plus flame haemorrhages, cotton wool spots or exudates.
4. Stage 3 plus papilloedema.

Note: Hypertension is associated with other vascular conditions such as retinal artery and vein occlusion and compounds complications of diabetic retinopathy.

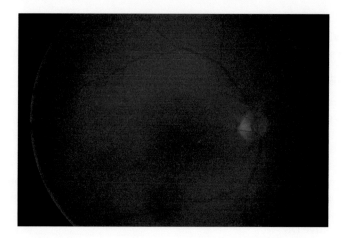

Figure 14.3 Arteriovenous nipping.

14.4 RETINAL VEIN OCCLUSION

Retinal vein occlusion (RVO) is the second most common retinal vascular disorder after diabetic retinopathy. Can be classified into the following.

- Central (CRVO) versus branch (BRVO): An occlusion at or proximal to the lamina cribrosa where the retinal artery exits the eye leads to CRVO (Figure 14.4). An occlusion of one of the branches of central retinal vein leads to BRVO (Figure 14.5).
- Ischaemic versus non-ischaemic.

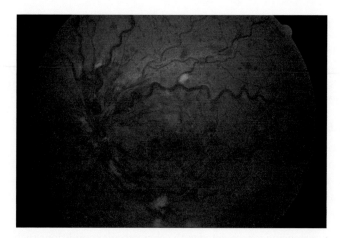

Figure 14.4 A central retinal vein occlusion.

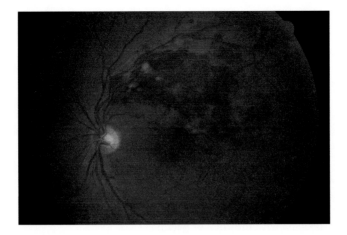

Figure 14.5 A branch retinal vein occlusion.

RISK FACTORS

- Age
- Microvascular: Hypertension, hyperlipidaemia and DM
- Combined oral contraceptive pill
- Glaucoma

CRVO

Non-ischaemic
- Sudden, painless dVA (>6/60).
- Fundoscopy: Tortuosity and dilatation of all branches of central retinal vein, dot/blot and flame haemorrhages of all four quadrants, prominent in the periphery, with optic disc and macular swelling.

Ischaemic
- Sudden, painless severe dVA (<6/60).
- Relative afferent pupillary defect (RAPD).
- Significant tortuosity and dilatation of all four quadrants with severe flame haemorrhages, disc and macular oedema.
- Rubeosis iridis in about 50% of patients, which can lead to NVG.

MANAGEMENT OF CRVO AS PER RCOPHTH (7)

Non-ischaemic
If VA is 6/96 or better and there is evidence of macular oedema on OCT:

- Commence intravitreal anti-VEGF or Ozurdex® (dexamethasone) implant).
- Both treatments are first line, although younger phakic patients or with history of glaucoma should be started on anti-VEGF. Patients with high cardiovascular profile should be started on Ozurdex implant.

Ischaemic

- No neovascularization and open angle: Monitor for neovascularization and glaucoma.
- Neovascularization present: Urgent PRP $\pm$ cyclodiode laser therapy if angle closure.

BRVO

- Most common location: Superotemporal, followed by inferotemporal.
- dVA, metamorphopsia, VF defect (altitudinal).
- Retinal haemorrhage in the affected quadrant.
- Complication: CMO and neovascularization.

MANAGEMENT OF BRVO AS PER RCOPHTH (7)

- Macular oedema with minimal ischaemia
    - Within 3 months of onset: Consider Ozurdex or anti-VEGF.
    - After 3 months of onset: Consider macular grid laser or Ozurdex or anti-VEGF.
- Macular oedema with marked ischaemia: No immediate treatment.
- Ischaemic BRVO with neovascularization: PRP.

14.5 RETINAL ARTERY OCCLUSION

Retinal artery occlusion (RAO) is an ophthalmic emergency. The most common cause is related to atherosclerosis. Other causes include giant cell arteritis (GCA).

CRAO

- Sudden painless loss of vision (VA usually counting fingers, unless cilioretinal is spared) with marked RAPD.
- Fundoscopy: Swollen, pale and opaque retina, 'cherry red' spot at the macula and arteriolar attenuation (Figure 14.6).

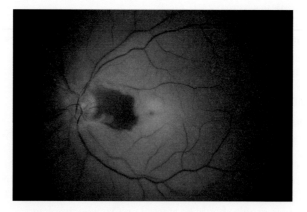

Figure 14.6 A central retinal artery occlusion with a 'cherry red' spot and arteriolar attenuation.

MANAGEMENT OF CRAO

Irreversible retinal infarction usually occurs within 90 minutes of occlusion of the artery, thus ocular massage, AC paracentesis and IOP-lowering interventions such as IV acetazolamide outside of this window have questionable efficacy.

BRANCH RAO (BRAO)

- Most commonly due to embolic causes.
- Sudden painless altitudinal field loss.
- Swollen white retina along the affected vessel with arteriolar attenuation (Figure 14.7).

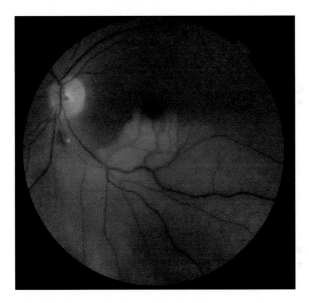

Figure 14.7 A branch retinal artery occlusion.

14.6 OCULAR ISCHAEMIC SYNDROME

Can be thought of as angina of the eye, with the majority of cases caused by atherosclerotic-stenosis of the carotid artery.

FEATURES

- Unilateral subacute dVA and periocular pain.
- Anterior segment: Conjunctival injection, AC cells and rubeosis iridis (IOP may remain low due to hypoperfusion).
- Posterior segment: Can be deceptively similar to CRVO. Cherry red macula, retinal artery attenuation and neovascularization of the disc are seen.

14.7 SICKLE CELL RETINOPATHY

Sickle cell anaemia is a blood disorder that affects the beta haemoglobin subunit of red blood cells (RBCs) and is more prevalent in patients of African-Caribbean origin.

When RBCs are exposed to hypoxia, they undergo a change in morphology resulting in a rigid, sickle-shaped cell. Intravascular sickling and haemolysis cause vascular occlusion and capillary nonperfusion, in both the anterior and posterior segment, leading to characteristic changes. Severity of ocular disease of different forms of sickle cell mutations is: HbSC > HbSThal > HbSS.

FEATURES

Sickle cell retinopathy can be either proliferative or nonproliferative:

- Nonproliferative: Includes signs of intraretinal haemorrhages ('salmon patches') or patches of RPE hyperplasia ('black sunbursts').
- Proliferative retinopathy (Goldberg classification [8]):
  1. Peripheral arteriolar occlusion
  2. Arteriovenous anastomosis
  3. Neovascularization with a 'sea fan' appearance
  4. Vitreous haemorrhage
  5. Tractional/rhegmatogenous retinal detachment

14.8 AGE-RELATED MACULAR DEGENERATION

Age-related macular degeneration (ARMD) is the leading cause of blindness in the elderly in developed countries. The disease process is limited to the macula of the eye, with large confluent soft drusen being the hallmark of the disease. Cell death in ARMD occurs through apoptosis.

PATHOLOGICAL CHANGES

Dry
- Drusen: Yellow deposits between Bruch's membrane and RPE (Figure 14.8).
- Atrophy of RPE, photoreceptor layers and choriocapillaries.
- Geographic atrophy: The end point of dry ARMD, characterized by large atrophic areas with visibility of underlying choroid (Figure 14.9).

Wet
- Ingrowth of choroidal vessels into RPE and subretinal space (choroidal neovascularization).
- Disciform macular degeneration is the end point of wet ARMD. This is fibrous scaring due to sub-RPE neovascularization (subretinal fibrosis).

Polypoidal choroidal vasculopathy (PCV)
- A variant of wet ARMD. Characterized by polypoidal dilatation of the choroidal vasculature. Progresses to subretinal haemorrhage and multiple PEDs.
- More common in middle-aged Asian populations and is unilateral in presentation.

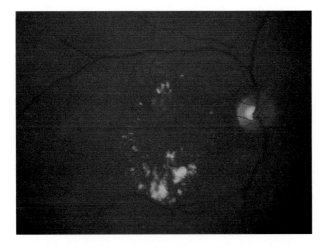

Figure 14.8 The drusen in dry age-related macular degeneration.

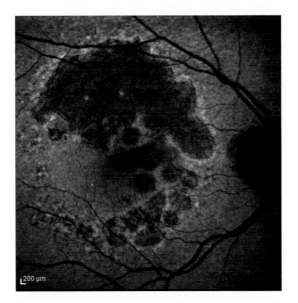

Figure 14.9 Geographic atrophy on autofluorescence angiography.

RISK FACTORS

- Increasing age: Most important risk factor
- Genetics: CFH and ARMS2 genes
- Smoking
- Hypermetropia
- Hypertension
- Female
- White race

FEATURES

Dry

- Gradual dVA and central scotoma.
- Intermediate or large soft drusen ($\geq$63 microns or $\geq$125 microns). *Note*: Small, hard drusen are of limited significance and may reflect normal age-related changes.
- Geographic atrophy of RPE.

Wet

- Decreased VA, metamorphopsia and central scotoma of sudden onset.
- Subretinal or sub-RPE haemorrhage and exudation.
- RPE and/or exudative retinal detachment.
- CMO.
- Subretinal fibrosis (disciform).

INVESTIGATIONS

- OCT: Most widely used test to monitor disease progress.
- ICG if PCV suspected: Branching vascular network may be seen on early frames, with hyperfluorescence of polyps in late frames.

MANAGEMENT

Dry

- Involves management of modifiable risk factors.
- Age-Related Eye Disease Study 2 (AREDS2) (9): Vitamin C, vitamin E, lutein, zeaxanthin and zinc proved to reduce the progression of ARMD. *Note*: Beta-carotene was removed as it increases the risk of lung cancer in smokers.
- AMSLER grid: To rule out progression to wet ARMD.

Wet

- Intravitreal anti-VEGF injections (e.g. ranibizumab or aflibercept).

Low vision aids

- Magnifiers: For reading, e.g. loop or spectacle magnifiers.
- Telescopes: For distance vision, e.g. Galilean telescopes.

14.9 CHOROIDAL NEOVASCULARIZATION (CNV)

Abnormal growth of vessels from the choriocapillaries through Bruch membrane into sub-RPE (type 1) or subretinal (type 2) space. Presentation of this disorder is with dVA, metamorphopsia and scotoma.

CAUSES

- Degenerative: ARMD (most common cause), myopic degeneration and angioid streak.
- Central serous chorioretinopathy.
- Inflammatory conditions: Birdshot choroidopathy, VKH, POHS.
- Best disease.
- Idiopathic.

14.10 DEGENERATIVE MYOPIA

Degenerative changes may occur in patients with progressive/pathological myopia. Those are a subset of patients with myopia $>-6D$ in which the axial length of the eye may never stabilize. It can be associated with Stickler, Marfan, Ehlers-Danlos and Down syndromes.

FEATURES

- Chorioretinal atrophy with visibility of underlying choroidal vessels.
- CNV.
- Rhegmatogenous retinal detachment.
- Macular hole.
- Posterior staphyloma
  - An outpouching of the posterior wall of the eye that has a different radius of curvature than the rest of the eye.
  - One of the hallmarks of pathological myopia, associated with poor prognosis.

14.11 ANGIOID STREAKS

Angioid streaks are usually bilateral symmetrical irregular atrophied streaks deep to the retina, radiating from the optic disc. These result from breaks in the Bruch membrane. The condition presents as peripapillary atrophy with multiple irregular streaks radiating in a circular pattern. (Figure 14.10). The most common cause of visual loss is CNV.

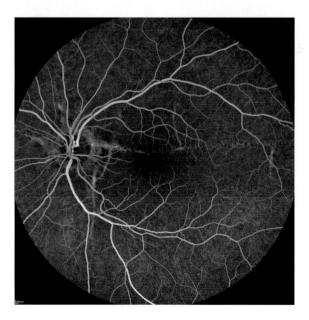

Figure 14.10 Agioid streaks on FA.

CAUSES

- Idiopathic.
- Pseudoxanthoma elasticum: Most common systemic association. Mutation in the ABCC6 gene. Presents with yellow papular lesions with excessive wrinkling ('plucked chicken' appearance) of skin usually in the neck, inguinal folds and antecubital fossa.
- Ehler-Danlos syndrome.
- Paget disease.

14.12 CYSTOID MACULAR OEDEMA

CMO is defined as retinal thickening of the macula due to abnormalities of the blood-retinal barrier which leads to leakage of fluid within the intracellular spaces of the retina, typically in the outer plexiform layer. Symptoms include dVA, metamorphopsia and scotoma. OCT is useful in detecting CMO and measuring retinal thickening (Figure 14.11).

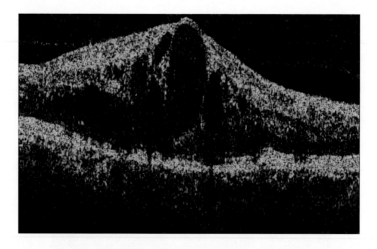

Figure 14.11 A cystoid macular oedema on OCT.

CAUSES

- Diabetic macular oedema
- CRVO and BRVO
- ARMD
- Uveitis typically pars planitis but also occurs in anterior and posterior uveitis
- Retinitis pigmentosa
- Irvine-Gass syndrome
- Drugs

14.13 CENTRAL SEROUS CHORIORETINOPATHY

Central serous chorioretinopathy (CSCR) refers to the buildup of central subretinal fluid due to retinal pigment epithelium dysfunction and choroidal hyperpermeability.

RISK FACTORS

- Males aged 20–50.
- Type A personality.
- Corticosteroid related: Iatrogenic or Cushing disease.

FEATURES

- Unilateral drop in VA, metamorphopsia, central scotoma.
- Slow recovery from bright light.
- Complications include serous (exudative) RD and CNV.

INVESTIGATIONS

- OCT: Triangle-shaped subretinal fluid collection with neurosensory retinal detachment (Figure 14.12).
- FA: Progressive leakage with 'inkblot' or 'smokestack' appearance.

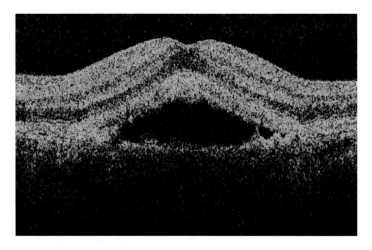

Figure 14.12 A central serous chorioretinopathy on OCT.

MANAGEMENT

- Observe (spontaneous resolution), with management of risk factors.
- Consider photodynamic therapy (verteporfin) when there is significant visual disturbance or chronic CSCR.

14.14 EALES DISEASE

Idiopathic peripheral retinal periphlebitis that typically occurs in young Indian males. Presentation is usually with recurrent vitreous haemorrhages. Tubercular protein exposure (tuberculin sensitivity) may be a risk factor for developing this disease.

14.15 BEST DISEASE

Best vitelliform macular dystrophy is an AD degeneration of the macula associated with lipofuscin accumulation in the RPE and atrophy of the photoreceptor layer of the retina.

FEATURES

- Bilateral condition associated with hypermetropic patients.
- Egg yolk lesion in macula: Yellow-orange circular elevated lesion (Figure 14.13).
- Electroretinogram (ERG): Normal.
- Electro-oculogram (EOG): Abnormal.
- Can be complicated by CNV which leads to dVA.

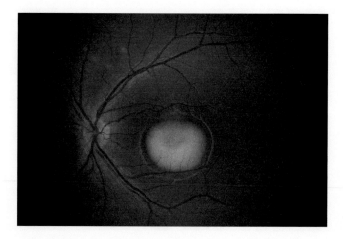

Figure 14.13 An egg-yolk lesion in Best disease.

14.16 STARGARDT DISEASE

An AR condition associated with a mutation in the ABCA4 gene on chromosome 1 that causes macular degeneration. Usually, it presents with reading difficulties in patients under 20.

SIGNS

- Normal-appearing fundus in early stages of the disease.
- Late fundal appearance
  - Beaten bronze appearance of the macula that can progress to geographic atrophy with a bull's-eye pattern.
  - Yellow-white flecks in RPE.
- FA: 'Dark choroid' (reduced choroidal circulation).

14.17 LEBERS CONGENITAL AMAUROSIS

An AR condition that presents with severe visual loss at birth, nystagmus and absent pupillary reflexes. Enophthalmos and subsequent keratoconus may occur due to constant rubbing of the eye (oculodigital syndrome). Fundoscopy findings are as follows.

- Early disease: Normal.
- Late disease: Salt-and-pepper retinopathy and bull's-eye maculopathy.

14.18 ALBINISM

Albinism is a hereditary group of diseases that affects melanin synthesis of the eye only (ocular albinism – XL inheritance) or, more commonly, the eye, skin and hair (oculocutaneous albinism – AR inheritance).

OCULAR FEATURES

- Symptoms: dVA due to foveal hypoplasia.
- Signs: Nystagmus, strabismus and iris/fundal hypopigmentation resulting in a 'pink eye' appearance.
- The optic chiasm contains more crossed fibres than normal.

14.19 RETINITIS PIGMENTOSA

A condition that is characterized by photoreceptor dysfunction (rods, then cones) and progressive atrophy/degeneration of retinal tissue. Most commonly due to a mutation in the rhodopsin gene in the long arm of chromosome 3. Inheritance can be AD (most common, least severe), AR or XL inheritance (worst prognosis).

FEATURES

- Symptoms: Nyctalopia (night blindness) and peripheral vision loss (tunnel vision in late disease).
- Triad: Pale optic disc (waxy disc) + bohny spicules + arteriolar attenuation (Figure 14.14).
- ERG (confirms diagnosis and monitors disease progression) and EOG are abnormal.

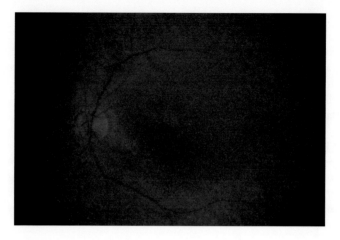

Figure 14.14 Retinitis pigmentosa.

ASSOCIATIONS

Optic disc drusen, myopia, posterior subcapsular cataract, CMO, open-angle glaucoma and keratoconus.

14.20 RETINITIS PIGMENTOSA-RELATED CONDITIONS

A group of AR conditions characterized by photoreceptor dysfunction with similar features to RP. All present with nyctalopia and tunnel vision with associated extraocular features.

USHER SYNDROME

- Most common inherited cause of combined deafness (sensorineural) + blindness.

REFSUM SYNDROME

- Accumulation of phytanic acid.
- Associated anosmia, peripheral neuropathy and ichthyosis.

BARDET-BIEDL SYNDROME

- RP-like retinopathy or bull's-eye maculopathy (cone-rod dystrophy more common).
- Associated learning disability, polydactyly and obesity.

BASSEN KORNZWEIG SYNDROME

- Abnormal absorption of fat-soluble vitamins.
- Associated spinocerebellar ataxia and acanthocytosis.

14.21 CAUSES OF LEUKOCORIA

Leukocoria is 'white pupil', or the absence of red reflex. Causes include:

- Congenital cataract
- Retinoblastoma
- Persistent fetal vasculature
- Retinopathy of prematurity (ROP)
- Coats' disease
- Toxocariasis

14.21.1 Retinoblastoma

Retinoblastoma is the most common primary intraocular malignancy in children. It arises from embryonal photoreceptor cells of the retina with a mutation in the tumour suppressor gene RB1 on the long arm of chromosome 13. Most commonly sporadic in inheritance but can be AD.

HISTOPATHOLOGY

Flexner rosettes are classic, but Homer-Wright rosettes and fleurettes may exist.

FEATURES AND DIAGNOSIS

- The average age of diagnosis is 3 years. Parents often notice loss of red reflex on photographs.
- Unilateral (sometimes bilateral) leukocoria + strabismus ± red eye and dVa.
- Funduscopy: White round mass with either endophytic (towards vitreous) or exophytic growth (towards RPE/choroid).
- Ultrasound scan (USS): Can show calcification with high internal reflectivity and can help determine tumour thickness.

14.21.2 Persistent fetal vasculature

Also known as persistent hyperplastic primary vitreous and is the failure of the fetal hyaloid vasculature to regress. This condition is associated with prematurity and development of cataract and retinal detachment. Patients present within the first 2 weeks of life with unilateral leukocoria, micro-ophthalmia and cataract (Mittendorf dot).

14.21.3 Retinopathy of prematurity

Blood vessels grow from the optic disc towards the periphery of the retina in utero, and this growth is driven through a relative hypoxic state. The main risk factor for the development of ROP is being born prematurely. The retinal vessels reach the nasal ora serrata (junction between retina and pars plana) at 32 weeks gestation and the temporal at 40 weeks. Hence, in ROP the temporal periphery is the first affected area (Figure 14.15).

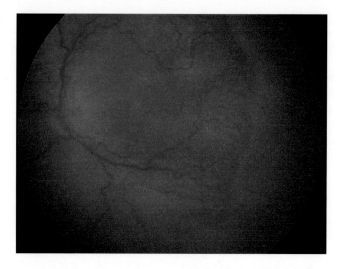

Figure 14.15 Retinal vessels not reaching the temporal periphery in retinopathy of prematurity.

RISK FACTORS

- Prematurely born infant (<32 weeks gestation).
- Weight less than 1500 g.
- Extended oxygen treatment; for example, in neonatal respiratory distress syndrome.

INTERNATIONAL CLASSIFICATION OF ROP REVISITED (10)

Location (Figure 14.16):
- Zone I: A circle with a radius of twice the distance from the disc to fovea with the optic disc being the centre.
- Zone II: Edge of zone I to nasal ora serrata.
- Zone III: From zone II to the remaining retina.

Stages
1. White demarcation line separating vascular from avascular areas.
2. Ridge: Elevated and thickened demarcation line (Figure 14.17).
3. Extraretinal fibrovascular proliferation or neovascularization infiltrating the vitreous.
4. Partial retinal detachment: (a) extrafoveal; (b) foveal.
5. Total retinal detachment (most commonly tractional).

Plus disease
Additional signs of increased venous dilatation and/or arteriolar tortuosity of the posterior retinal vessels can increase the severity of the condition.

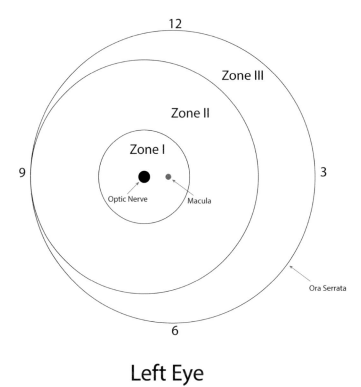

Figure 14.16 The zones of retinopathy of prematurity.

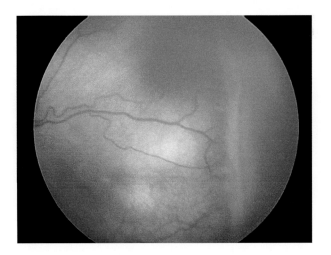

Figure 14.17 A stage 2 ridge in retinopathy of prematurity.

SCREENING

High-risk children should be screened via an indirect ophthalmoscope with 28D lens, as complications and permanent visual loss can occur if the disease is not treated early. UK ROP screening recommendations (11) include:

- All infants born at less than 32-weeks gestation and/or weighing less than 1501 g should be screened.
  - If born <27-weeks gestation, screen at 30–31 weeks postmenstrual age.
  - If born ≥27- and <32-weeks gestation *or* born >32-weeks gestational age but weigh <1501 g, screen after 4–5 weeks postnatal age.
- Screen weekly if stage 3 disease, plus disease or if vessels end at zone 1 or posterior zone 2. Otherwise, screen every 2 weeks.

MANAGEMENT

Treatment is usually within 48 hours with transpupillary diode laser. Treat if:

- Zone I, any stage with plus disease.
- Zone II, stage 3 with plus disease.
- Zone I, stage 3 without plus disease.

14.22 COATS' DISEASE

This is a unilateral condition of unknown aetiology that is characterized by telangiectasia and neovascularization. Commonly affects young boys.

FEATURES
- dVA, strabismus and leukocoria.
- Retinal telangiectasia and microaneurysms.
- Intra/subretinal exudation (Figure 14.18).
- Complications: Exudative retinal detachment and NVG.

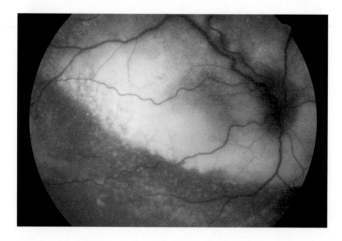

Figure 14.18 Telangiectasia and exudations in Coats' disease.

14.23 VON HIPPEL-LINDAU

AD condition affecting the von Hippel-Lindau (VHL) gene on the short arm of chromosome 3. This condition affects multiple organs including the brain, spinal cord, retina, kidneys, adrenal glands and pancreas.

FEATURES

- Retinal capillary haemangioma with tortuous feeder vessels
- Renal cell carcinoma
- Pheochromocytoma
- CNS haemangioblastoma

14.24 CHOROIDAL MELANOMA

Uveal tract malignant melanomas arise from melanocytes in either the iris, ciliary body or choroid. Choroidal melanoma is the most common. This tumour is usually unilateral in presentation and can be asymptomatic or cause dVA and exudative retinal detachment. They can appear pigmented (lipofuscin) with a 'collar-stud' configuration if Bruch's membrane is ruptured. Metastatic spread is usually to the liver. Chromosome 3 monosomy is an indicator of poor prognosis.

REFERENCES

1. Stratton IM, Adler AI, Andrew H, Neil W, Matthews DR, Manley SE et al. Association of glycaemia with macrovascular and microvascular complications of type 2 diabetes (UKPDS 35): Prospective observational study. *BMJ.* 2000;321(7258):405–12.
2. Diabetes Control and Complications Trial Research Group. The effect of intensive treatment of diabetes on the development and progression of long-term complications in insulin-dependent diabetes mellitus. *N Engl J Med.* 1993;329(14):977–86.
3. UK Prospective Diabetes Study Group. Tight blood pressure control and risk of macrovascular and microvascular complications in type 2 diabetes: UKPDS 38. *BMJ.* 1998;317(7160):703.
4. Diabetic Retinopathy Study Research Group. A modification of the Airlie House classification of diabetic retinopathy: Report 7. *Invest Ophthalmol Vis Sci.* 1981;21:210–26.
5. Early Treatment Diabetic Retinopathy Study Research Group. Grading diabetic retinopathy from stereoscopic color fundus photographs – An extension of the modified Airlie House classification: ETDRS report number 10. *Ophthalmology.* 1991;98(5):786–806.
6. The Royal College of Ophthalmologists. 2012. Diabetic Retinopathy Guidelines. https://www.rcophth.ac.uk/standards-publications-research/clinical-guidelines/
7. The Royal College of Ophthalmologists. 2015. Retinal Vein Occlusion Guidelines. https://www.rcophth.ac.uk/standards-publications-research/clinical-guidelines/

8. Goldberg MF. Natural history of untreated proliferative sickle retinopathy. *Arch Ophthalmol.* 1971;85(4):428–37.

9. Chew Emily Y, Clemons TE, SanGiovanni JP et al. Lutein+ zeaxanthin and omega-3 fatty acids for age-related macular degeneration: The Age-Related Eye Disease Study 2 (AREDS2) randomized clinical trial. *JAMA.* 2013;309(19):2005–15.

10. International Committee for the Classification of Retinopathy of Prematurity. The International Classification of Retinopathy of Prematurity revisited. *Arch Ophthalmol.* 2005;123:991–9.

11. RCPCH, RCOphth, BAPN, BLISS. Guideline for the screening and treatment of retinopathy of prematurity. 2008. https://www.rcophth. ac.uk/wp-content/uploads/2014/12/2008-SCI-021-Guidelines-Retinopathy-of-Prematurity.pdf

15

Vitreoretinal

MOSTAFA KHALIL AND OBAID KOUSHA

15.1 PERIPHERAL RETINAL DEGENERATION

These are abnormalities in the peripheral retina. Almost all individuals have some sort of abnormality in their peripheral retina. About 1 in 40 patients will develop retinal breaks associated with those abnormalities. A few important types are described below.

15.1.1 Lattice degeneration

These describe areas of thinning in the neurosensory retina (NSR) with overlying vitreous liquefaction and vitreoretinal adhesions, characterized by circumferential zigzag white lines with oval holes within the lesion. It is the most important degeneration predisposing to retinal tears. It is present in around 6–10% of the normal population and is more common in myopic eyes. Importantly, about 30% of patients with acute rhegmatogenous retinal detachment (RRD) have lattice degenerations (1). Prophylactic treatment should only be offered to those patients with a retinal detachment (RD) in the contralateral eye, in the form of laser retinopexy.

15.1.2 Degenerative retinoschisis

This is a microcystic degeneration resulting in the splitting of the retinal layers between the outer plexiform and inner nuclear layers, usually inferotemporally. It is a mostly bilateral and symmetrical condition. It is more common in hypermetropic eyes and is not frequently associated with RRD.

FEATURES

- Smooth convex and immobile elevation of retina with no demarcation line of chronicity as with RRD.
- Associated with absolute field defect.

15.2 POSTERIOR VITREOUS DETACHMENT

Posterior vitreous detachment (PVD) is the separation of the posterior vitreous cortex from the NSR. This occurs with increasing age as the vitreous becomes more liquefied (synchysis) which results in the creation of empty pockets of fluid within the vitreous, leading to vitreous collapse (syneresis). Eventually fluid escapes in the retrovitreous space separating the posterior hyaloid from the NSR (Figure 15.1). Six to eighteen percent of all patients presenting with an acutely symptomatic PVD could have a retinal tear. However, a PVD with vitreous haemorrhage is associated with a retinal tear in about 30–90% of patients (2).

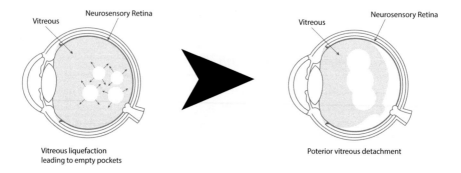

Figure 15.1 The formation of posterior vitreous detachment.

FEATURES

- Photopsia (light flashes) with associated floaters. VA usually not affected.
- Weiss ring: Thickened vitreous avulsed from optic disc.
- Shafer sign (pigmented particles or 'tobacco dust' in the anterior vitreous) negative.

MANAGEMENT

- Does not require treatment. Warn about risk of RRD and advise on presenting immediately if symptoms worsen or visual field affected.
- If complicated with retinal tear, treat with laser or cryoretinopexy.

15.3 RETINAL BREAKS

These are full-thickness retinal defects. Progression to RD is rare. Only treat when there is high risk of RD:

- High myopia >6D
- Aphakia
- Giant retinal tear
- Symptomatic U-shaped retinal tear
- Systemic disease (e.g. Stickler syndrome)

Several types exist, as follows.

RETINAL TEAR

A U-shaped defect due to anterior vitreoretinal traction on a strip of retina due to PVD (Figure 15.2). Can be associated with vitreoretinal adhesions such as at the margins of lattice degenerations. Progression to RRD occurs in a third of cases. Features include flashes, floaters, Weiss ring and Shafer sign positive. All symptomatic U-shaped retinal tears should be treated with laser retinopexy.

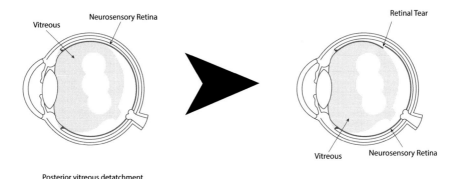

Figure 15.2 The formation of a retinal tear from vitreoretinal traction caused by posterior vitreous detachment.

GIANT RETINAL TEAR

A retinal tear extending ≥3 clock hours (≥90°). Location: Peripheral retina at posterior border of vitreous. Associated with PVD, as are retinal tears. Bilateral in 16.5% of cases, with retinal tears in the fellow eye in 60% of patients. Associations include trauma, high myopia, diseases (e.g. Marfan or Stickler syndrome). Management is with laser retinopexy for both eyes.

RETINAL DIALYSIS

A disinsertion of the retina at the ora serrata involving anterior and posterior to the vitreous base. Traumatic retinal dialysis is more common and located superonasally. Idiopathic dialysis is more commonly located inferotemporally. Retinal dialysis is the leading cause of traumatic RD in children and young adults. Management is with laser retinopexy if there is no associated RD, otherwise scleral buckle is used.

15.4 RETINAL DETACHMENT

RD is the separation of the NSR from the RPE. Following this, there is subsequent shift of subretinal fluid (SRF), called shifting SRF, in the space between the NSR and the RPE. Three main types of retinal detachment exist: RRD, tractional RD and exudative RD.

15.4.1 Rhegmatogenous retinal detachment

Rhegmatogenous is the most common form of retinal detachment and occurs due to a retinal break. Fluid seeps in between the NSR and RPE causing a detachment (Figure 15.3). This is an emergency – it can lead to blindness if left untreated.

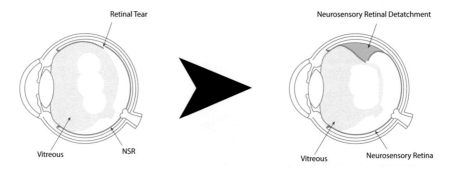

Figure 15.3 The formation of a retinal detachment from a previous retinal tear.

FEATURES
- Flashes and floater.
- Curtain-like visual field loss (relative field loss).
- dVA if macula is involved.
- RAPD, Weiss ring and Shafer sign.
- Presence of PVD and retinal breaks (commonly a U-shaped retinal tear; most common location is superotemporal).
- Fresh RRD
  - Convex and corrugated dome-shaped surface with loss of RPE markings (Figure 15.4).

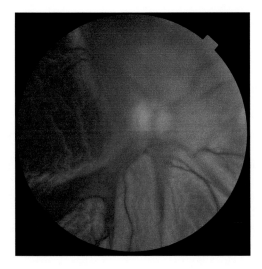

Figure 15.4 A fresh rhegmatogenous retinal detachment.

- Shape based on most superior retinal break.
- Extend from ora serrata to optic disc.
- They are progressive and may affect macula.
- Chronic RRD (Figure 15.5)

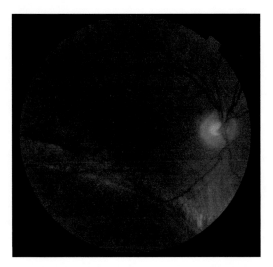

Figure 15.5 An old rhegmatogenous retinal detachment.

- Retinal thinning.
- Demarcation lines.
- Intraretinal cysts.
- Proliferative vitreoretinopathy.

INVESTIGATIONS

- Slit lamp biomicroscopy with wide-field lens.
- Indirect ophthalmoscopy with scleral depression to visualise the ora serrata.
- B-scan USS if there is no view of posterior pole such as dense cataract or vitreous haemorrhage.

MANAGEMENT

There is variation among surgeons on which surgery to choose. For simplicity:

- Vitrectomy: Most commonly used procedure, indicated for posterior retinal breaks, giant retinal tears and proliferative vitreoretinopathy.
- Scleral buckle: Very high success rate. Used in simple RRD and retinal dialysis when there is no pre-existing PVD.
- Pneumatic retinopexy: Lower success rate but also fewer side effects; used in carefully selected cases with small superior breaks 1 clock hour apart between 11 and 1 clock hours.

15.4.2 Tractional retinal detachment

This type of retinal detachment is due to vitreoretinal traction. This is an insidious process where fibrovascular membranes cause progressive contracture over areas of adhesions eventually causing a detachment. The most common causes are advanced proliferative diabetic retinopathy and ROP.

FEATURES

- Usually asymptomatic (no flashes or floaters), as there is no PVD.
- VA affected once macula is threatened, causing distortion of vision.
- Detachment: Shallow immobile concave tenting of retina.
- Minimal shifting SRF.
- Associated relative visual field loss, signs of underlying disease.

MANAGEMENT

- Vitrectomy with membrane peel.

15.4.3 Exudative retinal detachment

This rare form of RD occurs due to buildup of SRF from damage to the outer blood-retinal barrier. Fluid leakage occurs under the retina thereby separating the NSR from the RPE. This occurs when the compensatory mechanisms of the RPE fail to pump the fluid back into the choroidal circulation.

AETIOLOGY

- Tumours: Choroidal tumours.
- Idiopathic: Nanophthalmia leading to uveal effusion syndrome.
- Vascular: Exudative age-related macular degeneration, Coats' disease, central serous chorioretinopathy.

- Inflammatory
  - Posterior uveitis: Sympathetic ophthalmia and VKH.
  - Posterior scleritis, orbital inflammatory disease, postop inflammation and extensive pan-retinal photocoagulation.

FEATURES

- Floaters if vitritis present, dVA if macula is affected.
- RD: Smooth convex that is shallow or bullous. Lack of PVD and retinal tears and evidence of traction.
- Evidence of underlying condition.

MANAGEMENT

- Ophthalmic and systemic history and examination including blood pressure and urinalysis.
- Treatment of underlying cause treats the retinal detachment; surgery not usually indicated.

15.5 VITREOUS HAEMORRHAGE

This is bleeding into the vitreous chamber. May be due to two basic mechanisms: rupture of vessels through trauma or bleeding from pathological processes.

CAUSES

- Trauma
  - Blunt or penetrating trauma causing closed or open globe injury.
  - Shaken baby syndrome.
  - Acute PVD-associated with vitreous haemorrhage.
- Neovascularization leading to haemorrhage
  - Diabetic retinopathy.
  - Sickle cell retinopathy.
  - ROP.
  - Wet ARMD.
  - Retinal vein occlusion.
- Other: Choroidal tumours.

INVESTIGATION

- All patients need a detailed fundal examination to assess the severity of haemorrhage and exclude retinal tears.
- Indirect ophthalmoscopy aids in visualization of the peripheral retina.
- B-scan USS to exclude retinal tears.

MANAGEMENT

- Management is directed depending on the cause.
- Pan-retinal photocoagulation if there is a fundal view.
- Intravitreal anti-VEGF if there is no fundal view or in wet ARMD.

- Pars plana vitrectomy, often pre-treated with intravitreal anti-VEGF, for non-clearing vitreous haemorrhage or in presence of retinal detachment.

15.6 CHOROIDAL DETACHMENT

A detachment of the choroid from the sclera due to the accumulation of fluid or blood in the suprachoroidal space.

AETIOLOGY

- Acute hypotony (IOP <5 mmHg), typically following glaucoma surgery.
- Trauma.

FEATURES

- Smooth, dark and convex elevation arising from the periphery.
- Large 'kissing' choroidal detachments can lead to RD.

15.7 CHOROIDAL RUPTURE

A break in the choroid may result from closed globe injury due to blunt trauma. There is usually disruption of the choroid, Bruch membrane and RPE; however, the neurosensory retina is unaffected. On examination, a crescent-shaped yellow subretinal streak is seen usually adjacent to the optic disc.

15.8 UVEAL EFFUSION SYNDROME

This is a rare and bilateral abnormality of the choroid and sclera. It is most commonly seen in middle-aged hypermetropic males and is associated with nanophthalmos (axial length <20 mm).

FEATURES

- Mild inflammation
- Thickened sclera
- Ciliochoroidal detachment
- Exudative RD
- RPE hypertrophic areas ('leopard spots') in chronic cases

MANAGEMENT

- Full-thickness sclerotomies.

15.9 EPIRETINAL MEMBRANE

This is an avascular fibrocellular sheet or membrane that develops on the surface of the retina. It is more common in female patients. These arise from proliferation of RPE, glial cells or hyalocytes on the surface of the retina. Contracture on the retina leads to problems such as elevation of the retina and CMO.

SYNONYMS

- In appearance: Cellophane maculopathy, macular pucker.
- In pathogenesis: Premacular fibrosis, idiopathic premacular gliosis.

CAUSES

- Idiopathic
- Trauma
- Posterior uveitis
- BRVO
- Iatrogenic (cryotherapy, photocoagulation, retinal detachment surgery)

FEATURES

- Asymptomatic.
- Metamorphopsia and dVA.
- Cellophane membrane: May be transparent, best seen with red-free light (look for glistening light reflex).
- Macular pucker: Thick contracted membrane with mild distortion of blood vessels.
- Other findings: Macular pseudohole, CMO, retinal haemorrhages and telangiectasia.

INVESTIGATIONS

- OCT.

MANAGEMENT

- Observation: Is an option if the condition is stable.
- Vitrectomy.

15.10 MACULAR HOLE

A full-thickness defect in the fovea with splitting of all neurosensory retinal layers from the internal limiting membrane to the RPE. This condition is a common cause of central visual loss in females aged 60–70.

CAUSES

- Primary: Vitreous traction on the fovea from a PVD (vitreomacular traction).
- Secondary: Does not have vitreomacular traction. For example, cases caused by trauma or high myopia.

FEATURES

- Metamorphopsia with central dVA.

CLASSIFICATION

Used to be classified by the 'Gass classification' (3); however, this has been replaced by the OCT classification, 'International Vitreomacular Traction Study (IVTS) classification' (4) (Table 15.1).

Table 15.1 Macular hole classification

IVTS classification	Gass classification
Vitreomacular adhesion	–
Vitreomacular traction (VMT) (Figure 15.6)	Stage 1: Impending macular hole with loss of foveal depression
Small or medium macular hole with VMT	Stage 2: Small full-thickness macular hole (<400 microns)
Medium or large macular hole with VMT	Stage 3: Large full-thickness macular hole (≥400 microns)
Small, medium or large macular hole without VMT	Stage 4: Full-thickness macular hole with PVD evidenced by a Weiss ring (Figure 15.7)

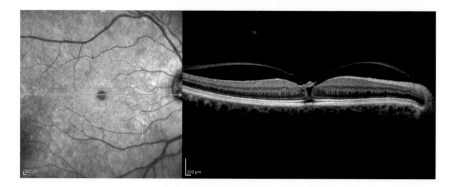

Figure 15.6 A vitreomacular traction.

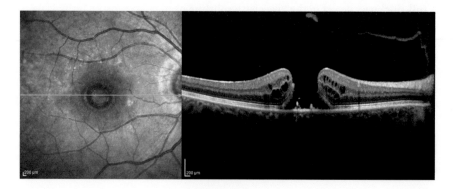

Figure 15.7 A full-thickness macular hole.

MANAGEMENT

- Usually, patients are observed in stage 1.
- Stage 2 macular holes can be managed with either vitrectomy or intravitreal vitreolysis with ocriplasmin.
- Stages 3 and 4 can be managed with vitrectomy, internal limiting membrane peel and gas tamponade.

15.11 HEREDITARY VITREORETINAL DEGENERATIONS

These are rare congenital conditions characterized by early retinal and vitreal degeneration. There are many types of these degenerations. X-linked retinoschisis, Stickler syndrome and Wagner syndrome are discussed here.

15.11.1 X-linked retinoschisis

Note that X-linked retinoschisis is different from degenerative retinoschisis, which is discussed under peripheral retinal degenerations. X-linked retinoschisis is due to intercellular adhesion abnormalities which lead to splitting of the retina at the nerve fibre layer.

FEATURES

- Typically presents in early childhood: Hypermetropic boys present with reading difficulties at primary school.
- On examination: Bilateral maculopathy, foveal schisis with spoke-like folds with cystoid changes. Resembling CMO without leakage on FA.

INVESTIGATION

- Scotopic ERG (-ve ERG): Normal a wave, loss of b wave with oscillatory potentials.

15.11.2 Stickler syndrome

Stickler syndrome is the most common inherited cause of RD. This condition is AD and occurs due to a defect in collagen synthesis (mainly type II).

FEATURES

- Ophthalmic: High myopia, cortical cataracts, ectopia lentis, glaucoma, optically empty vitreous, radial lattice-like retinal degeneration and RRD.
- Sensorineural deafness.
- Pierre Robin features: Micrognathia, glossoptosis, cleft palate, flat nasal bridge and maxillary hypoplasia.
- Marfanoid features.

MANAGEMENT

- Prophylactic 360° retinal laser.
- Vitrectomy if RD occurs.

15.11.3 Wagner syndrome

This AD disorder is similar to Stickler syndrome but without the systemic features.

FEATURES

- Low myopia
- Cortical cataracts
- Optically empty vitreous

RD is linked to this condition but is less common than in Stickler syndrome and so they are treated if they occur (not prophylactically).

REFERENCES

1. Lewis H. Peripheral retinal degenerations and the risk of retinal detachment. *Am J Ophthalmol.* 2003;136(1):155–60.
2. Sarrafizadeh R, Hassan TS, Ruby AJ, Williams GA, Garretson BR, Capone A Jr et al. Incidence of retinal detachment and visual outcome in eyes presenting with posterior vitreous separation and dense fundus-obscuring vitreous hemorrhage. *Ophthalmology.* 2001;108(12):2273–8.
3. Gass J, Donald M. Idiopathic senile macular hole: Its early stages and pathogenesis. *Arch Ophthalmol.* 1988;106(5):629–39.
4. Duker JS, Kaiser PK, Binder S, De Smet MD, Gaudric A, Reichel E et al. The International Vitreomacular Traction Study Group classification of vitreomacular adhesion, traction, and macular hole. *Ophthalmology.* 2013;120(12):2611–9.

Ocular trauma

MOSTAFA KHALIL, OMAR KOULI AND RIZWAN MALIK

16.1 LEFORT FRACTURES

LEFORT I

Horizontal fracture of the maxilla. The fracture passes through the alveolar ridge of the upper teeth, lateral nose and the walls of maxillary sinus.

LEFORT II

Fracture through the medial wall of maxilla, inferior orbital rim, nasal and lacrimal bones and through or near the infraorbital foramen.

LEFORT III

Fracture passes through the nasofrontal and frontomaxillary sutures, ethmoid air cells, and zygomatic arch.

16.2 ORBITAL FLOOR FRACTURE

An indirect blowout fracture to the orbital floor is commonly caused by a rapid increase in intraorbital pressure leading to compression of the globe posteriorly and a fracture of the orbital floor, typically the maxillary bone.

FEATURES

- Eyelids: Ecchymosis (racoon eyes) and oedema.
- Vertical diplopia: Entrapment of the IR muscle causes inability to upgaze. Children can develop oculocardiac syndrome, which is a drop in heart rate with movement of the extraocular muscles. This may lead to cardiac arrest in extreme circumstances.
- Hypoesthesia over the distribution of the infraorbital nerve.
- Enophthalmos.

INVESTIGATIONS

- Visual function tests and acuity should be examined.
- Hess charts: To examine and monitor eye movements.
- CT scans: Show a 'teardrop' sign in cases of soft tissue prolapse in the maxillary antrum (Figure 16.1).

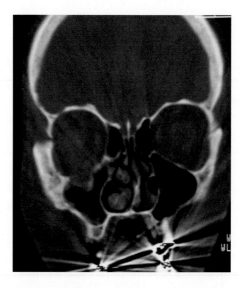

Figure 16.1 Right orbital floor fracture with a 'teardrop' sign.

MANAGEMENT

- Observation to allow swelling to subside.
- Surgical repair for persistent diplopia.

16.3 INTRAOCULAR FOREIGN BODIES

Intraocular foreign bodies (IOFB) are common and may be present following open globe injuries. The most toxic IOFB are copper and contaminated organic material. Important to note that penetrating trauma cannot be excluded even if there are no entry wounds on examination.

EXAMINATION

- Both eyes must be examined even if the other eye is asymptomatic.
- Examination of the eyelids for any lacerations.
- Fluorescein drops are helpful to determine the site of injury, and a slit lamp examination can be used.
- Funduscopy: Assess the posterior segment.

INVESTIGATIONS

- CT: To detect the IOFB and its location. It is considered superior to an x-ray, as x-rays are less able to detect radiolucent materials (e.g. glass). However, x-rays can be used to rule out IOFB.
- MRI: Contraindicated in metallic IOFB.

MANAGEMENT

- Prophylactic antibiotics such as systemic ciprofloxacin. In cases of contaminated IOFB, intravitreal antibiotics (vancomycin + ceftazidime) are considered.
- Surgical removal with the use of magnets or forceps.

COMPLICATIONS

- Sympathetic ophthalmia in the fellow eye.
- Endophthalmitis.
- Angle recession glaucoma.
- Red cell glaucoma.

16.4 CHEMICAL INJURY

Chemical injuries can either be alkali or acidic. Alkali materials are lipophilic and are more destructive due to their penetrative potential. Acidic causes coagulation of the surface protein impeding their own progression. One exception, however, is hydrofluoric acid, which can rapidly penetrate the eye.

FEATURES

- Severe pain, lacrimation and dVA.
- Lid oedema.
- Conjunctiva: Epithelial loss, injection chemosis, ischaemia (eye may look 'white and quiet' due to severe ischaemia), necrosis.
- Cornea: Epithelial damage, oedema, necrosis.
- Anterior chamber: Flare, mydriasis, increased IOP.
- Limbal ischaemia is useful to assess prognosis.

MANAGEMENT

- Irrigation: Should be done immediately before any examination is performed. Test the pH, then instill topical anaesthetic and irrigate with water.

- Topical/oral antibiotics + topical steroids + cycloplegia + preservative-free artificial tears must be given.
- For more severe injuries, early surgery is necessary.

16.5 SHAKEN BABY SYNDROME

Also called abusive head trauma; commonly presents with multilayered retinal haemorrhages in children under the age of 2 years. Associated with irritability, vomiting and cerebral bleeds.

16.6 PURTSCHER RETINOPATHY

Usually bilateral disease originally described in association with severe trauma. Can be seen in association with acute pancreatitis (Purtscher-like retinopathy). Presents with sudden painless dVA, cotton wool spots, Purtscher flecken (areas of retinal whitening) and haemorrhages.

Questions & Answers

OMAR KOULI AND MOSTAFA KHALIL

PAPER 1: QUESTIONS

1. Which of the following is not a management option for macular hole?
   a. Pars plana vitrectomy with internal limiting membrane peel
   b. Observation
   c. Intravitreal vitreolysis ocriplasmin
   d. PRP
2. Which part of the retina is suppressed in exotropia in order to avoid diplopia?
   a. Temporal
   b. Nasal
   c. Inferior
   d. Superior
3. Which of the following increases the risk of retinal detachment?
   a. Hypermetropia
   b. Microphthalmia
   c. Postop rise in IOP
   d. Preop PRP
4. Which slit lamp illumination technique is used to view corneal endothelium?
   a. Direct illumination
   b. Diffuse illumination
   c. Specular reflection
   d. Indirect illumination (retroillumination)
5. Which low vision aid can help a patient with ARMD watch TV?
   a. Loop magnifier
   b. Galilean telescope
   c. Hubble telescope
   d. Magnifying glasses

6. How many layers are in the retina?
   a. 10
   b. 5
   c. 2
   d. 9

7. A Turkish male admits to having recurrent oral and genital ulcers. He presents with a painful red eye. What is the diagnosis?
   a. Reiter syndrome
   b. Bechet disease
   c. Toxoplasmosis
   d. Birdshot choroidopathy

8. What HLA is birdshot choroidopathy associated with?
   a. HLA-B5
   b. HLA-DR5
   c. HLA-A29
   d. HLA-B27

9. A young myopic male presents with blurred vision on exertion. Mid-peripheral spoke-like iris transillumination defects are seen. What is the diagnosis?
   a. Pseudoexfoliation syndrome
   b. Pigment dispersion syndrome
   c. Angle recession glaucoma
   d. NVG

10. Which of the following is correctly matched?
   a. Blunt trauma and shield-like cataract
   b. Atopic dermatitis and flower-shaped cataract
   c. Myotonic dystrophy and snowflake cataract
   d. Wilson disease and sunflower cataract

11. A female patient presents with painful eye movements, dyschromatopsia, dVA, and leg weakness. A spinal MRI shows continuous signal abnormalities in three vertebral segments. What is the diagnosis?
   a. Lyme disease
   b. Cat scratch disease
   c. Multiple sclerosis
   d. Neuromyelitis optica

12. A male with type A personality presents with central vision loss and metamorphopsia. OCT shows a triangular-shaped subretinal fluid with neurosensory retinal detachment. Which of the following is the diagnosis for the above scenario?
   a. CSCR
   b. Macular hole
   c. Eales disease
   d. Irvine-Gass syndrome

13. A contact lens wearer presents with severe ocular pain. Perineural and ring-shaped corneal stromal infiltrates are seen. What is the diagnosis?
    a. Bacterial keratitis
    b. Filamentary keratitis
    c. Fungal keratitis
    d. *Acanthamoeba* keratitis

14. A mother notices that her 2-year-old's eyes are white in a photograph. Bilateral loss of red reflex is seen on ophthalmoscopy. What is the likely cause?
    a. Retinoblastoma
    b. Congenital cataract
    c. Toxocariasis
    d. Coats' disease

15. What muscle is most commonly affected in TED?
    a. IR
    b. MR
    c. SO
    d. LR

16. A patient with T2DM presents with gradual dVA and metamorphopsia. Fundoscopy and OCT confirmed the diagnosis. What is the management?
    a. PRP
    b. Intravitreal anti-VEGF
    c. ETDRS macular laser
    d. PPV

17. Which retinal detachment is most likely in a patient with severe proliferative diabetic retinopathy?
    a. Rhegmatogenous
    b. Exudative
    c. Tractional
    d. None of the above

18. A disinsertion of the retina at the ora serrata is a description of which of the following?
    a. Retinal dialysis
    b. Retinal tear
    c. PVD
    d. Retinal detachment

19. Which of the following causes inferior altitudinal defect?
    a. Non-arteritic AION
    b. Occipital lobe lesion
    c. CRAO
    d. Temporal lobe lesion

20. What is the most common cause of central scotoma?
    a. Multiple sclerosis
    b. ARMD
    c. Nutritional optic neuropathy
    d. Glaucoma

21. Which of the following drugs causes CMO?
    a. Chloramphenicol
    b. Latanoprost
    c. Ethambutol
    d. Hydroxycholoroquine

22. Which of the following drugs causes bull's-eye maculopathy?
    a. Chloramphenicol
    b. Latanoprost
    c. Ethambutol
    d. Hydroxycholoroquine

23. Which of the following charts can be used to assess VA of a child <1 years old?
    a. Keeler cards
    b. Kay pictures
    c. Sheridan Gardner
    d. LogMAR

24. Which of the following diseases is not included in the Vision 2020 Global Initiative?
    a. Onchocerciasis
    b. Retinoblastoma
    c. Trachoma
    d. Cataract

25. Which of the following are incorrectly matched?
    a. Craniopharyngioma and bitemporal hemianopia
    b. Tilted disc and superotemporal field defect
    c. Calcarine artery occlusion and homonymous hemianopia with macular sparing
    d. Temporal radiation lesion and inferior homonymous quadrantopia

26. A patient presents with anisocoria. The right eye has absent pupillary response to light. The near reflex is strong but with slow re-dilatation. What is the diagnosis?
    a. Horner syndrome
    b. Adie's pupil
    c. Parinaud syndrome
    d. Argyll Robertson

27. Which of the following pass through the cavernous sinus?
    a. CNVI
    b. CNIII
    c. CNIV
    d. CNV

28. Which of the following is not proven to slow myopic progression?
    a. Outdoor activity
    b. Using atropine drops
    c. Using reading glasses
    d. None of the above
29. Which of the following is true about von Hippel-Lindau?
    a. Associated with meningioma
    b. Associated with retinal capillary haemangioma
    c. Genetic mutation on chromosome 6
    d. Diagnosed in the sixth decade
30. Which ocular structure has the highest refractive power?
    a. Lens
    b. Vitreous humour
    c. Aqueous humour
    d. Cornea
31. An obese female complains of morning headaches and momentary loss of vision. Enlarged blind spots are seen on fundoscopy. What is the diagnosis?
    a. Migraine
    b. Postural hypotension
    c. Papilloedema
    d. Amaurosis fugax
32. Damage to what structure causes downbeat nystagmus?
    a. Pons
    b. Vestibulocerebellum
    c. Dorsal midbrain
    d. Hypothalamus
33. CNIII passes between which arteries?
    a. Inferior cerebral and anterior cerebellar
    b. Superior cerebellar and posterior cerebral
    c. Inferior cerebellar and posterior cerebral
    d. Superior cerebral and anterior cerebellar
34. Which of the following does not cause leukocoria?
    a. ROP
    b. Coats' disease
    c. Eales disease
    d. Toxocariasis
35. What is the most common cause of inherited combined deafness and blindness?
    a. Usher syndrome
    b. Refsum disease
    c. Retinitis pigmentosa
    d. Alport syndrome
36. Which of the following is caused by vigabatrin toxicity?
    a. Binasal hemianopia
    b. Bitemporal hemianopia
    c. Central scotoma
    d. Junctional scotoma

37. What collagen type is found in the sclera?
    a. I
    b. II
    c. III
    d. IV

38. What chromosome is HLA found on?
    a. Long arm of chromosome 9
    b. Short arm of chromosome 6
    c. Short arm of chromosome 9
    d. Long arm of chromosome 6

39. What MRI finding is seen in patients with TED?
    a. MR muscle enlargement with tendon sparing
    b. LR muscle enlargement with tendon sparing
    c. MR muscle and tendon are typically enlarged
    d. MRI is normal in TED

40. What is used to blanch vascular congestion seen in episcleritis?
    a. Apraclonidine
    b. Timolol
    c. Pilocarpine
    d. Phenylephrine

41. Which of the following is the least likely pathology in TED?
    a. Overstimulation of Müller muscle
    b. LR-restrictive myopathy
    c. MR-restrictive myopathy
    d. Levator palpebrae-restrictive myopathy

42. Which of the following is not an intervention for myopic correction?
    a. Peripheral corneal ablation with LASIK
    b. Negative diopter lens
    c. Central corneal ablation with LASIK
    d. Central corneal ablation with LASEK

43. Which of following is true about the lens?
    a. The lens becomes more spherical when looking at a distance.
    b. The posterior capsule thickens with age.
    c. The anterior suture has an inverted Y shape.
    d. The posterior suture has an inverted Y shape.

44. Which of the following will not interfere with IOP measurement?
    a. Excessive pressure on eyelids by examiner
    b. Low CCT
    c. Astigmatism
    d. Timolol use

45. Which of the following is true about LogMAR?
    a. The number of letters increases as you move down the chart.
    b. The letter spacing is equal to one letter width.
    c. A LogMAR of +1 is equal to a Snellen score of 6/6.
    d. A LogMAR of 0 is equal to a Snellen score of 6/60.

46. Which of the following is false about LogMAR?
    a. The row spacing is equal to the height of a letter from the row below.
    b. The letter size increases in 0.1 LogMAR steps.
    c. Each letter can be assigned a score of 0.01.
    d. There are five letters on each line.

47. Which of the following is false regarding functional visual loss?
    a. Presentation is with dVA and is more common in females.
    b. Tunnel vision is seen.
    c. Optokinetic nystagmus is absent.
    d. Normal pupils with no RAPD.

48. Which of the following is false regarding photoreceptors?
    a. There is a 20:1 ratio of rods:cones.
    b. Rods contain the pigment iodopsin.
    c. Cones form a 1:1 ratio with bipolar cells.
    d. The wavelength of maximum absorbance of rods is 498 nm.

49. Which of the following bones make up the medial orbital wall?
    a. Zygomatic, ethmoidal, lacrimal, frontal
    b. Zygomatic, ethmoidal, lacrimal, maxilla
    c. Maxillary, ethmoidal, lacrimal, lesser wing of sphenoid
    d. Maxillary, ethmoidal, lacrimal, greater wing of sphenoid

50. Surgery for unilateral congenital cataract should be performed within what time period?
    a. 6 weeks
    b. 8–10 weeks
    c. 10–12 weeks
    d. No treatment (spontaneous resolution)

51. Which of the following does not travel through the common tendinous ring?
    a. CNIII
    b. CNIV
    c. CNVI
    d. Nasociliary branch of CNV_1

52. A 4-month-old infant with a 30PD esotropia has cross fixation on a cover test, and a horizontal jerky nystagmus moving away from the covered eye. What is the diagnosis?
    a. Infantile esotropia
    b. Microtropia
    c. Basic esotropia
    d. Convergence excess esotropia

53. Which of the following is false regarding microtropia?
    a. Squint angle is usually <10PD.
    b. Amblyopia is common.
    c. Microtropia is associated with anisometropia in most of the cases.
    d. Microtropia with identity moves on cover testing.

54. Which of the following is not a cause of bitemporal hemianopia?
    a. Bilateral internal carotid aneurysm
    b. A large anterior communicating artery aneurysm
    c. Pituitary adenoma
    d. Craniopharyngioma
55. Which of the following is false regarding congenital glaucoma?
    a. There is a triad of tearing, blepharospasm and photophobia.
    b. It is associated with buphthalmos and Haab striae.
    c. It is usually unilateral.
    d. It is more common in boys.
56. Which of the following is associated with HLA-DR5?
    a. VKH
    b. Juvenile idiopathic arthritis
    c. Sympathetic ophthalmia
    d. Birdshot choroidopathy
57. Which of the following does not cause vision loss in juvenile idiopathic arthritis?
    a. Glaucoma
    b. Band keratopathy
    c. CMO
    d. Optic atrophy
58. Which of the following is the first-line treatment for ROP?
    a. PRP
    b. Anti-VEGF
    c. Transpapillary diode laser
    d. Vitrectomy
59. Which of the following regarding TED are incorrectly matched? (2 answers)
    a. Dalrymple sign and lid lag on downgaze
    b. Von Graefe sign and lid lag on downgaze
    c. Von Graefe sign and lid retraction
    d. Dalrymple sign and lid retraction
60. Which of these is associated with CD4+ counts <50?
    a. Herpes simplex
    b. CMV
    c. Toxoplasmosis
    d. Toxocariasis
61. Which of the following is not a test for stereopsis?
    a. Titmus test
    b. Lang test
    c. Frisby test
    d. Bagolini glasses

62. Which EOM is unlikely to be affected following retrobulbar anaesthetic block?
    a. LR
    b. IO
    c. SO
    d. IR

63. A patient presents with 1 mm anisocoria in both light and dark. What is the likely diagnosis?
    a. Parinaud syndrome
    b. Argyll Robertson
    c. Physiological anisocoria
    d. Adie's pupil

64. What is the management of CSCR?
    a. PRP
    b. Anti-VEGF
    c. Dexamethasone implant
    d. Photodynamic therapy

65. Calcium deposition in band keratopathy occurs in which corneal layer?
    a. Bowman
    b. Endothelium
    c. Descemet
    d. Epithelium

66. Which of the following is not part of the driving criteria for cars?
    a. At least 6/12 vision
    b. Able to see car registration plate at 18 metres
    c. At least 120° of horizontal visual field
    d. Controlled diplopia

67. Which of the following fits the severely sight impaired criteria?
    a. VA <3/60 with full visual field
    b. VA 3/60–6/60 with full visual field
    c. VA 6/60–6/24 with moderate reduction of visual field
    d. VA ≥6/24 with homonymous hemianopia

68. Which of the following is not associated with calcification?
    a. Retinoblastoma
    b. Toxocariasis
    c. Band keratopathy
    d. Toxoplasmosis

69. What type of hypersensitivity is associated with trachoma?
    a. I
    b. II
    c. III
    d. IV

70. Which of the following is true regarding indirect ophthalmoscopy?
    a. A +20D concave lens is required.
    b. The field of illumination is largest in myopia.
    c. The image is virtual.
    d. The image is erect.

71. A patient presents with pulsatile proptosis, whooshing sound and conjunctival chemosis post-trauma. What is the diagnosis?
    a. Neuroblastoma
    b. Direct CCF
    c. Indirect CCF
    d. Cavernous sinus thrombosis

72. 'Cobblestone' papillae superiorly in the conjunctiva and Horner-Trantas dots are typical of which condition?
    a. *Acanthamoeba* keratitis
    b. Viral conjunctivitis
    c. VKC
    d. Trachoma

73. Which of the following does not typically occur at the outer plexiform layer?
    a. CMO
    b. Hard exudates
    c. Dot blot haemorrhages
    d. Microaneurysms

74. In which condition are Flexner rosettes found?
    a. Retinoblastoma
    b. Neuroblastoma
    c. Medulloblastoma
    d. Rhabdomyosarcoma

75. The following are AD inheritance except:
    a. Best disease
    b. Refsum disease
    c. Neurofibromatosis
    d. Stickler syndrome

76. Pulmonary artery aneurysm is pathogenomic of:
    a. Behçet disease
    b. Kawasaki disease
    c. Vogt-Koyanga-Harada syndrome
    d. Tenson syndrome

77. Colour vision is tested using:
    a. N-type
    b. Cardiff
    c. TNO
    d. Ishihara chart

78. Which of the following is used to differentiate a postganglionic from a preganglionic lesion in Horner syndrome?
    a. Cocaine drops
    b. Adrenaline
    c. Hydroxyamphetamine
    d. Atropine drops
79. A lesion in the right MLF will cause:
    a. Failure of abduction in the left eye
    b. Failure of adduction in the left eye
    c. Failure of abduction in the right eye
    d. Failure of adduction in the right eye
80. What percentage of PVD with associated vitreous haemorrhage have retinal tears?
    a. Not associated
    b. 5–15%
    c. 15–30%
    d. 30%
81. Which of the following is not associated with infantile esotropia?
    a. Dissociative vertical deviation
    b. Myopia
    c. IO overaction
    d. Latent nystagmus
82. Which of the following is not a complication of refractive eye surgery?
    a. Diffuse lamellar keratitis ('Sands of Sahara syndrome')
    b. Dry eyes
    c. PCO
    d. Glare
83. Which of the following is not associated with myopia?
    a. Congenital glaucoma
    b. RRD
    c. Uveal effusion syndrome
    d. ROP
84. Which of the following is not a complication of PRP?
    a. Retinal detachment
    b. Vitreous haemorrhage
    c. Peripheral visual loss
    d. CMO
85. Which of the following is not involved in pupillary constriction?
    a. Edinger-Westphal
    b. CNIII
    c. Ciliospinal centre of Budge
    d. Pretectal nucleus

86. Which of the following is used to manage keratoconus?
    a. LASIK
    b. LASEK
    c. Toric lenses
    d. Rigid contact lenses
87. Which of the following regarding contact lenses is used in patients with dry eyes?
    a. Silicone hydrogel
    b. Monthly lenses
    c. Soft lenses
    d. Rigid lenses
88. Which of the following genes is associated with Stargardt?
    a. ABCA4
    b. COL2A1
    c. Rhodopsin
    d. CFH
89. Which of the following is associated with HLA-B51?
    a. Kawasaki
    b. Behçet disease
    c. Reiter syndrome
    d. Multiple sclerosis
90. Which of the following is used to treat onchocerciasis?
    a. Mebendazole
    b. Pyrimethamine
    c. Ivermictin
    d. Coamoxivlav

PAPER 1: ANSWERS

1d	19a	37a	55c	73d
2a	20b	38b	56b	74a
3b	21b	39a	57d	75b
4c	22d	40d	58c	76a
5b	23a	41b	59a + c	77d
6a	24b	42a	60b	78c
7b	25d	43d	61d	79d
8c	26b	44d	62c	80b
9b	27a	45b	63c	81b
10d	28c	46c	64d	82c
11d	29b	47c	65a	83c
12a	30d	48b	66b	84d
13d	31c	49c	67a	85c
14b	32b	50a	68b	86d
15a	33b	51b	69d	87a
16b	34c	52a	70b	88a
17c	35a	53d	71b	89b
18a	36a	54a	72c	90c

PAPER 2: QUESTIONS

1. An elderly woman presents with headaches, diplopia that is worse on distance and esotropia in the primary position. What is the likely diagnosis?
   a. Consecutive esotropia
   b. CNVI palsy
   c. Simple esotropia
   d. Distance exotropia

2. What is the size of the adult eye?
   a. 17 mm
   b. 24 mm
   c. 28 mm
   d. 34 mm

3. A patient presents with a headache and neck pain. On examination, you find a left ptosis and miosis. What is the likely diagnosis?
   a. Internal carotid dissection
   b. Posterior communicating artery aneurysm
   c. Anterior communicating artery aneurysm
   d. Uncal herniation

4. A 20-year-old male was involved in an RTA. A few hours later he is found asleep and unarousable. He has a fixed dilated pupil, hypertension and bradycardia. What is the likely diagnosis?
   a. Uncal herniation
   b. Subarachnoid haemorrhage
   c. Horner syndrome
   d. Subdural haemorrhage

5. What ocular condition is associated with tuberose sclerosis?
   a. Optic nerve glioma
   b. Optic nerve meningioma
   c. Retinal astrocytoma
   d. Retinal haemangioma

6. A patient suffers blunt trauma to the eye. Which of the following is unlikely to occur?
   a. Angle recession glaucoma
   b. NVG
   c. Hyphema
   d. Orbital floor fracture

7. A patient presents with dVa, floaters and painful red eye 5 days post-phacoemulsification. What is the likely causative organism?
   a. *Staphylococcus aureus*
   b. *Streptococcus viridians*
   c. *Staphylococcus epidermidis*
   d. *Propionibacterium acnes*

8. Where is the genetic abnormality in von Hippel-Lindau?
   a. Short arm of chromosome 3
   b. Long arm of chromosome 17
   c. Short arm of chromosome 12
   d. Long arm of chromosome 22

9. A patient with ophthalmoplegia is only able to abduct the right eye. What is the likely diagnosis?
   a. One-and-a-half syndrome
   b. Intranuclear ophthalmoplegia
   c. CNVI palsy
   d. Carotid dissection

10. A patient with diabetic maculopathy is treated with anti-VEGF injections. What is the best investigation to monitor the maculopathy?
    a. FA
    b. Ishihara charts
    c. OCT
    d. B-scan ultrasound

11. Which of the following is used to distinguish between open- and closed-angle glaucoma?
    a. Gonioscopy
    b. Tonometry
    c. Perimetry
    d. Fundoscopy

12. Which of the following is not a side effect of acetazolamide?
    a. Metabolic acidosis
    b. Paraesthesia
    c. Renal stones
    d. Optic neuritis

13. A patient presents with sudden-onset dVA and RAPD. They have a swollen pale retina and arteriolar attenuation. What is the likely diagnosis?
    a. CRAO
    b. Ischaemic optic neuropathy
    c. Severe DR
    d. Amaurosis fugax

14. What is associated with superior limbic keratoconjunctivitis?
    a. Trachoma
    b. TED
    c. Tolosa-Hunt syndrome
    d. Idiopathic orbital inflammation

15. What is the first sign seen in DR?
    a. Microaneurysms
    b. Arteriolar narrowing
    c. Cotton wool spots
    d. Dot haemorrhages

16. A patient with vertical gaze palsy, frequent falls and parkinsonism is typical of what?
    a. Multiple system atrophy
    b. Friedreich ataxia
    c. Progressive supranuclear palsy
    d. Cerebellar stroke

17. A homeless man develops bilateral centrocaecal scotoma. He is also found to have macrocytic anaemia. What is the likely diagnosis?
    a. Kjer's optic neuropathy
    b. Nutritional optic neuropathy
    c. Leber's optic neuropathy
    d. Sickle cell retinopathy

18. A corneal flap is created, the stroma is then ablated, and the flap is replaced. What is this a description of?
    a. PRK
    b. LASIK
    c. LASEK
    d. YAG laser capsulotomy

19. When is the IOP highest?
    a. Morning
    b. Night
    c. Unchanged
    d. Midday

20. Which of the following is true regarding BCC?
    a. Peripheral palisading cells are present.
    b. It is more common in the upper eyelid.
    c. There is lymphatic metastasis.
    d. It enlarges aggressively over a few weeks.

21. How long should soft contact lenses be withheld for before undergoing laser eye surgery?
    a. 7–14 days
    b. 14–21 days
    c. 21–28 days
    d. 28–35 days

22. A patient presents with a hyphema following trauma. When will a secondary bleed be likely to occur?
    a. 3–7 days
    b. 1–3 days
    c. 14–21 days
    d. After 28 days

23. Which of the following is an incorrect statement?
    a. OCT uses infrared radiation.
    b. ICG has high permeability when passing through the choroid.
    c. ICG angiography is particularly useful at visualizing the choroid.
    d. Autofluorescence uses lipofuscin present in the RPE.

24. What nerve is likely to be affected in a patient with ectropion, dry eye and reduced facial expressions?
    a. CNVII
    b. CNIII
    c. CNX
    d. CNV$_1$

25. What is the visual acuity of a newborn?
    a. 6/24
    b. 6/200–6/60
    c. 6/60
    d. 6/18–6/6

26. Which of the following tests is used to test the visual acuity of an 18-month-old child?
    a. Cardiff cards
    b. Kay pictures
    c. Sheridan-Gardiner
    d. LogMAR

27. Which of the following controls smooth pursuit?
    a. Frontal lobe
    b. Thalamus
    c. Temporal lobe
    d. Occipital lobe

28. What investigation is used to measure corneal curvature?
    a. Keratometry
    b. Tonometry
    c. Perimetry
    d. Pachymetry

29. When the angle of incidence is greater than the critical angle:
    a. Total internal reflection occurs.
    b. Total external refraction occurs.
    c. Reflection mostly occurs with some refraction.
    d. The angle of incidence cannot be greater than the critical angle.

30. Which of the following is true regarding ophthalmoscopy?
    a. The image is real and inverted.
    b. It provides stereoscopic vision.
    c. An area of 4 disc diameters is viewed.
    d. It provides ×15 magnification.

31. Which of the following are pairs of yoke muscles?
    a. Left SO and right SR
    b. Left LR and right MR
    c. Right IO and left LR
    d. Right SR and left IR

32. When does the eye reach its maximum axial length?
    a. 3–7 years old
    b. Does not stop growing
    c. 13–18 years old
    d. 1–3 years old

33. Which of the following structures is affected leading to presbyopia?
    a. Cornea
    b. Iris
    c. Zonules
    d. Lens

34. Which of the following retinal cells is involved in light pupillary response?
    a. Ganglion cells
    b. Ciliary ganglion
    c. Bipolar cells
    d. Photoreceptor cells

35. Corneal stroma originates from the:
    a. Neural ectoderm
    b. Mesoderm
    c. Neural crest
    d. Surface ectoderm

36. RPE originates from the:
    a. Neuroectoderm
    b. Mesoderm
    c. Neural crest
    d. Surface ectoderm

37. Which of the following leads to a highest risk of PCO?
    a. Acrylic hydrophobic lens
    b. PMMA
    c. Silicone oil
    d. Acrylic hydrophilic lens

38. Which of the following contains multinucleated cells on biopsy?
    a. Giant cell arteritis
    b. Neurofibromatosis
    c. Retinoblastoma
    d. Choroidal melanoma

39. Kocher sign is seen in which of the following?
    a. Myasthenia gravis
    b. Orbital inflammatory disease
    c. TED
    d. Neuroblastoma

40. What is the most common cause of blindness worldwide?
    a. ARMD
    b. Trachoma
    c. Vitamin A deficiency
    d. Cataracts

41. What is the most common cause of childhood blindness in Africa?
    a. Refractive errors
    b. Trachoma
    c. Vitamin A deficiency
    d. Retinopathy of prematurity
42. What is the most common cause of axial proptosis?
    a. Neuroblastoma
    b. Rhabdomyosarcoma
    c. Orbital cellulitis
    d. TED
43. *Onchocerca volvulus* is transmitted to humans via:
    a. Cat
    b. *Simulium* black fly
    c. Dog
    d. Mosquito
44. Ophthalmic lasers are under which laser safety class?
    a. 1–2
    b. 2
    c. 3a–3b
    d. 3b-4
45. A reduction of 1% in HbA1c reduces the progression of diabetic retinopathy by:
    a. 10%
    b. 5%
    c. 37%
    d. 26%
46. A child presents with a superficial red lesion on his upper eyelid that enlarges on crying. What is the likely diagnosis?
    a. Capillary haemangioma
    b. Port wine stain
    c. Choroidal haemangioma
    d. Cavernous haemangioma
47. A child with learning disability presents with seizures and port wine stain. What ophthalmic condition is associated?
    a. Capillary haemangioma
    b. Choroidal haemangioma
    c. Retinal astrocytoma
    d. Lich nodules
48. A patient presents with yellow papular lesions with excessive wrinkling in their neck and axilla described as 'plucked chicken' skin. Which of the following is associated with this disease?
    a. Lich nodules
    b. Retinal astrocytoma
    c. Angioid streaks
    d. Retinal haemangioma

49. A patient suffers blunt trauma to the eye. Fundoscopy shows a crescent-shaped yellow subretinal streak concentric to the optic disc. What is the likely diagnosis?
    a. Angioid streaks
    b. Choroidal melanoma
    c. Choroidal rupture
    d. PVD

50. Choroidal melanomas commonly metastasize to:
    a. Brain
    b. Liver
    c. Bone
    d. Lungs

51. What is the management of toxoplasmosis?
    a. Sulfadiazine
    b. Ivermictin
    c. Mebendazole
    d. Immunoglobulin

52. Which of the following antibiotics affects nucleic acid synthesis?
    a. Penicillin
    b. Tetracyclines
    c. Fluoroquinolones
    d. Vancomycin

53. Which of the following light wavelengths can cause photokeratitis?
    a. Ultraviolet
    b. Infrared
    c. Visible light
    d. X-rays

54. Which of the following is absorbed by haemoglobin and melanin only?
    a. Frequency-doubled Nd:YAG
    b. Argon blue-green
    c. PRP
    d. Diode laser

55. Which of the following causes vortex keratopathy?
    a. Amiodarone
    b. Tetracycline
    c. Chloramphenicol
    d. Vigabatrin

56. Which of the following organisms is associated with the worst prognosis in endophthalmitis?
    a. *Bacillus cereus*
    b. *Staphylococcus epidermidis*
    c. *Staphylococcus aureus*
    d. *Propionibacterium acnes*

57. Which of the following is a correct statement regarding IOP?
    a. A thick CCT underestimates IOP.
    b. Excessive fluorescence does not affect IOP measurements.
    c. Excessive pressure on the eyelid overestimates IOP.
    d. Astigmatism does not affect accuracy of IOP measurements.
58. Regarding marijuana and IOP, which of the following is correct?
    a. It increases IOP.
    b. It decreases IOP for approximately 36 hours.
    c. Tachyphylaxis can occur.
    d. It has no effect on IOP.
59. Excessive skin of the upper eyelid leading to ptosis that occurs in elderly patients is referred to as:
    a. Neurofibroma
    b. Blepharophimosis, ptosis and epicanthus inversus syndrome (BPES)
    c. Dermatochalasis
    d. Blepharochalasis
60. Which foramen does the nerve that supplies sensory innervation to the skin below the eye exits the orbit?
    a. Superior orbital fissure
    b. Foramen rotundum
    c. Infraorbital foramen
    d. Jugular foramen
61. The sympathetic fibres for pupillary dilation pass through the:
    a. Edinger-Westphal nucleus
    b. Pretectal nucleus
    c. Carotid canal
    d. Ciliary ganglion
62. A child presents with rapidly progressive unilateral proptosis. which of the following needs to be ruled out?
    a. Rhabdomyosarcoma
    b. Neuroblastoma
    c. Lymphangioma
    d. Cavernous haemangioma
63. What is the likely diagnosis in a diabetic patient presenting with sudden painless loss of vision one week after cataract surgery?
    a. PCO
    b. Endophthalmitis
    c. CMO
    d. CRVO
64. A diabetic man is admitted to the ICU with sepsis. He later develops dVA and floaters. Fundoscopy shows multiple white creamy retinal lesions in his right eye. What is the likely causative organism?
    a. Herpes simplex
    b. CMV
    c. Candida
    d. *Acanthamoeba*

65. Where is the prevalence of multiple sclerosis highest in the UK?
    a. Scotland
    b. England
    c. Wales
    d. Northern Ireland

66. A patient with ptosis and muscle fatigability is typical of which condition?
    a. Guillain-Barre syndrome
    b. Myasthenia gravis
    c. Lambert-Eaton syndrome
    d. Miller Fisher syndrome

67. A tumour associated with NF1 and shows fusiform enlargement of the optic nerve on CT is called:
    a. Optic nerve glioma
    b. Optic nerve sheath meningioma
    c. Optic nerve haemangioma
    d. Craniopharyngioma

68. An African patient presents with dVA. Fundoscopy shows multiple arteriovenous anastomosis. What is the likely diagnosis?
    a. Sickle cell retinopathy
    b. Hypertensive retinopathy
    c. DR
    d. Wet ARMD

69. A patient with a headache has a fixed dilated pupil with ptosis. What is the likely cause?
    a. Anterior communicating artery aneurysm
    b. Carotid dissection
    c. Posterior communicating artery aneurysm
    d. Internal carotid aneurysm

70. Bitot spots are seen in:
    a. Xerophthalmia
    b. Sjögren syndrome
    c. Sickle cell retinopathy
    d. Trachoma

71. Which extraocular muscle inserts closest to the limbus?
    a. SR
    b. IR
    c. MR
    d. LR

72. Which of the following tests sensory fusion?
    a. Bagolini glasses
    b. Titmus
    c. TNO
    d. Prisms

73. Which of the following is most likely to cause night blindness?
    a. Cone-rod dysfunction
    b. Rod-cone dysfunction
    c. Coats' disease
    d. Retinoblastoma

74. A patient with presbyopia says he can now see without his reading glasses. Which cataract does the patient have?
    a. Posterior subcapsular
    b. Nuclear sclerotic
    c. Cortical
    d. Anterior subcapsular

75. What is the investigation of choice for orbital cellulitis?
    a. MRI
    b. X-ray
    c. Ultrasound
    d. CT

76. Where is the lesion in a patient with an incongruous left homonymous superior quadrantopia?
    a. Right temporal radiation
    b. Left parietal radiation
    c. Right parietal radiation
    d. Left temporal radiation

77. Which interleukin produces CRP?
    a. IL-5
    b. IL-12
    c. IL-6
    d. IL-8

78. Number of cases of a disease in a particular population at a particular time is a description of:
    a. Incidence
    b. Prevalence
    c. Specificity
    d. Sensitivity

79. The ability of a test to correctly identify individuals who do not have a disease is a description of:
    a. Incidence
    b. Prevalence
    c. Specificity
    d. Sensitivity

80. Which of the following is used to grow *Acanthamoeba*?
    a. Chocolate agar
    b. Lowenstein Jensen medium
    c. Non-nutrient *Escherichia coli* agar
    d. Meat broth

81. Which of the following is true regarding saccades?
    a. Slow movements
    b. Long lasting (>100 milliseconds)
    c. Initiation of voluntary saccades occurs in the contralateral frontal eye field
    d. PPRF controls vertical saccades

82. What muscle is commonly entrapped in orbital floor fractures?
    a. IR
    b. MR
    c. IO
    d. LR

83. Which of the following is incorrect regarding the image formed by prisms?
    a. Virtual
    b. Erect
    c. Diminished
    d. Displaced towards the apex

84. Ectopia lentis in Marfan syndrome is usually:
    a. Nasal
    b. Superotemporal
    c. Inferonasal
    d. Inferior

85. A lesion in which of the following would not cause an RAPD?
    a. Retina
    b. Anterior optic tract
    c. Optic radiation
    d. Optic chiasm

86. A child presents with a retinal detachment. He has high myopia, optically empty vitreous, micrognathia and a flat nasal bridge. What is the likely diagnosis?
    a. Stickler syndrome
    b. X-linked retinoschisis
    c. Wagner syndrome
    d. Choroidal detachment

87. What is the likely causative organism of cannaliculitis?
    a. *Streptotoccus pneumoniae*
    b. Pseudomonas
    c. *Actinomyces israelii*
    d. *Haemophilus influenzae*

88. Which of the following is used to suture the iris?
    a. Silk
    b. Polyglactin 910
    c. Nylon
    d. Polypropylene

89. Where is the neurosensory retina derived from?
    a. Outer cup of diencephalon
    b. Inner cup of diencephalon
    c. Outer cup of telencephalon
    d. Inner cup of telencephalon
90. A fracture that involves the nasal, lacrimal and medial maxillary wall is called?
    a. Lefort I
    b. Lefort II
    c. Lefort III
    d. Lefort IV

PAPER 2: ANSWERS

1b	19a	37b	55a	73b
2b	20a	38a	56a	74b
3a	21b	39c	57c	75d
4a	22a	40d	58c	76a
5c	23b	41c	59c	77c
6b	24a	42d	60c	78b
7c	25b	43b	61c	79c
8a	26a	44d	62a	80c
9a	27d	45c	63c	81c
10c	28a	46a	64c	82a
11a	29a	47b	65a	83c
12d	30d	48c	66b	84b
13a	31b	49c	67a	85c
14b	32c	50b	68a	86a
15a	33d	51a	69c	87c
16c	34a	52c	70a	88d
17b	35c	53a	71c	89b
18b	36a	54a	72a	90b

Index

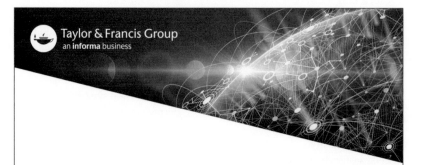